Daniel Peter Layard

An essay on the bite of a mad dog

Daniel Peter Layard

An essay on the bite of a mad dog

ISBN/EAN: 9783337814939

Printed in Europe, USA, Canada, Australia, Japan

Cover: Foto ©ninafisch / pixelio.de

More available books at **www.hansebooks.com**

AN ESSAY

ON THE

BITE

OF A

MAD DOG.

By DANIEL PETER LAYARD, M. D.

Phyſician to Her Royal Highneſs the Princeſs Dowager of WALES, Member of the Royal College of Phyſicians in LONDON, and of the Royal Society.

Conveniens homini eſt, hominem ſervare voluptas,
Et melius nulla quæritur arte favor.

OVID. Epiſt.

The SECOND EDITION.

LONDON:

Printed for JOHN RIVINGTON, in St. Paul's Church-yard; and THOMAS PAYNE, at the Mews-gate.

MDCCLXIII.

Sir EDWARD WILMOT,

BARONET, M. D.

Fellow of the Royal College of Phyficians in LONDON, and of the Royal Society, Firft Phyfician to His Moft Sacred MAJESTY, and Phyfician General to the Army.

SIR,

TO reverence patrons while living, and to hold their memory in the higheft veneration after this life, is the duty of every open hearted and grateful mind.

The publication of this Effay, affords me the favorable opportunity of expreffing in the ftrongeft manner, my gratitude for the unmerited favors I re-

ceived

ceived from that no lefs gene-
rous and humane MÆCENAS,
than learned and fuccefsful
phyfician Doctor MEAD.

Like many others, at my
firft fetting out in practice, I
found in him an encourager,
who far from fupercilioufly de-
fpifing the inabilities and want
of experience in youth, felt a
pleafure in animating and in-
citing them to cultivate that
emulation and zeal, which by
their application they fhewed
for the ftudy of whatever might
prove ufeful.

The benevolent friend to
mankind, in this as in other
inftances, ftrictly adhered to
his MOTTO, and proved that he
was formed   NON

Non sibi, sed toti.

Accept Sir of this imperfect
work, as a token of that re-
spectful remembrance I shall
ever retain for Doctor Mead,
and of my true regard for all his
family.

That You, Sir, whom two
succeeding monarchs have highly honored and deservedly dis-
tinguished, may continue to
enjoy the royal confidence and
the full possession of whatever
you can desire, is the hearty
and sincere wish of

Sir,

Your most obedient and

most obliged humble Servant,

London March
28, 1762.
Daniel Peter Layard.

THE
PREFACE.

WHENEVER a calamity of any kind befalls fociety, it is natural for every individual to join in the alarm, and to enquire into the means of leffening, or avoiding the danger.

The fubject of the following effay, although examined and treated of, by many authors of the moft refpectable character, is of too near and general concern for mankind to remain fatisfied with the doubtful and apprehenfive ftate in which they were left, through the uncertain effects of the cures hitherto directed. Many remedies have proved fuccefsful, which in other conftitutions or climates failed. And the

only

only method to be depended upon feemed of too recent a date, for the univerfal adoption of that practice, without a confirmation of it's utility by repeated facts.   It therefore behoved
every one, whofe profeffion was the
healing art, to examine into the particular nature of this difeafe, the reafons why it had been fo long undeter-
mined in it's qualities and cure, and
to remove fuch prejudices as were the
ftrongeft obftacles to fuch a defirable
end.

Notwithftanding the higheft veneration and moft fincere refpect was paid
to Doctor MEAD's effay on this fubject,
yet the later improvements of others,
deferved alfo their due confideration;
and fome fuccefsful cures incited me,
not only to examine into the manner
of their being performed, but alfo upon a clear conviction of the method being advantageous, I have ventured to
ftate the facts and illuftrate the difcoveries of others, by bringing the account

count of this fo terrifying difeafe to the teft of reafon ; for as CELSUS obferves in his preface, the practice of medicine ought to be rational.

This effay in the introduction, endeavors to fhew, that the fmall advances in the knowlege of this difeafe, and the uncertainty of it's cure are owing to common prejudices and vulgar errors, which have always proved of the greateft hinderance to the progrefs of every fcience, but particularly of the art and practice of medicine.—And alfo it points out the nature of this diftemper incident to mankind, from the bite of a mad dog.

The firft fection treats of the bite of a mad dog, as the caufe of the malady, examines into the properties of the *faliva* of thofe animals, and by what means it becomes hurtful and poifonous to other creatures. The progrefs of this poifon is alfo traced, and it's various effects enquired into.

Doctor

Doctor MEAD's fyftem, that the nervous fluid is chiefly affected in this difeafe, has been called in queftion, and
the nerves themfelves have been fixed
upon as the feat of this diftemper, and
all the fymptoms accounted for by the
fpafmodic contractions of the nerves. I
have induftrioufly avoided all unprofit-
able controverfies, which in the art of
medicine, as in all other arts and fci-
ences, tend more to divide than to reconcile and convince the difputants.
It probably may be in this cafe, as in
many others, that by yielding and mak-
ing fome allowances on each fide, truth
would be eafier afcertained than by ca-
villing through motives of pride and
obftinacy. The wife father of phyfic
has told us*, *That our art is extenfive,
and our life but fhort.* Why fhould
we then wafte in trifling and needlefs
altercations the little time we have to
run over the vaft field of medicine ?

---

* HIPPOCRATIS Aphorifm i.

Men

Men of the greatest abilities and acknowleged underſtandings have acquieſced
in the perſuaſion of a nervous fluid,
and of it's being not only the agent of
the ſoul, but alſo that it is liable to be
deſtroyed or propagated. Thoſe who
deny it's exiſtence, do not refuſe to acknowlege that the nerves are compoſed of a prolongation of the *meninges*, containing a pulpous portion of the
brain, or *cerebellum*, *medulla oblongata*,
or *medulla ſpinalis* in them, but will
not allow that the nerves are vaſcular,
and therefore ſolve all their actions by
the vibrations, oſcillations, and ſpaſ-
modic contractions of the nerves. Allowing theſe external effects, which
BAGLIVI, and the later accurate experiments of profeſſors HALLER and WHYTT,
and of Doctor BROCKLESBY, plainly
evince of the irritability of the nervous
parts, why may not the opinions of
thoſe learned profeſſors and Doctors,
SYDENHAM, BAGLIVI, BORELLUS, BO-
ERHAAVE, MEAD, HOFFMANN, LIEU-
TAUD,

TAUD, WHYTT, and HUXHAM in favor of a nervous fluid, or animal fpirits be adopted ? And at the fame time
that we find in thofe authors the proof
of a *ftimulus* in the blood, which acts
on the nervous fibres of the blood-veffels, why may not the exiftence of a
fentient voluntary principle be allowed
of, which directs our will and motions
at the fame time that the component
particles of the blood, particularly the
falts, ftimulate the veffels to fuch a degree, as to preferve the circulation of
the ftreams of life ? If it be urged that
no one ever difcovered either the nervous fluid or the veffels the animal fpirits pafs through, may it not be an-
fwered ? That the OMNIPOTENT CRE-
ATOR has framed thofe tubes according to their ufe, and notwithftanding
they may be too fine for our difcovery
even with the beft microfcopes, yet it
may not be contrary to common reafon, that they may be fo formed as to
convey proper fubtile, elaborated particles

ticles from our blood, which may ferve as the different links of the chain which connects our intellectual and corporeal faculties together; the exiftence of which rational foul intimately connected with our body, no one will prefume to deny, although the means whereby they are united are effectually hidden from our limited view. How ftrenuoufly foever both fides may feem to infift on their different opinions, it is very evident that their purfuit in practice, are the fame; both in food and medicine, time out of mind, fuch diet or phyfic has been given, which would promote the greateft feparation of active particles to increafe the fpirits; and even thofe who ftimulate the nerves, to produce their contractions, adminifter, and apply the fame remedies to augment the circulation and heat, which is conftantly leffened by perfpiration. Since whatever be the fingular notions of each fide, they both follow the fame intentions,

there

there can neither be fatisfaction nor u-
tility in taking part in the difpute, but
every one is to be left to enjoy his own
opinion.

The fecond fection enquires into the
hydrophobia, and fhews that this affrighting fymptom is common to other
difeafes, although not fo general or peculiar, as in this one, occafioned by
the bite of a mad dog.

The third fection examines the feveral methods of cure, whether rational or empirical. Among others,
bathing in the fea, or in cold fpring
water, are feverally treated of. I have
freely given my opinion in relation to
every external application, or internal
medicine, ufed for the cure of this difeafe, and have endeavored particularly
to fhew that Doctor MEAD's powder,
although far from being an infallible
remedy, is neither ufelefs, or void of
merit. In the confideration of the different methods which are recommended, I have had conftantly before me
the

the example set to every physician by professor BOERHAAVE and Doctor MEAD. It is well known by many, and recorded by Doctor MATY, who was intimately acquainted with both, that those learned men were not always of the same opinion, and yet their emulation towards the improvement of their profession was so disinterested and void of jealousy, that they retained for each other the highest sense of esteem and friendship; never were displeased with each other when they differed in opinion, but mutually and reciprocally communicated their observations and designs, and were constantly presenting one another with tokens of their regard. This humane and benevolent turn of mind in them both, appears in Doctor MATY's characters of those two great men *. And he instances, that

* Essai sur le caractere du Grand Medecin, ou eloge critique de Mr. BOERHAAVE.
Journal Britannique, tom. xiv. Ann. 1754, mois de Juillet & Aout article 1er. p. 229, 230. Eloge du Docteur RICHARD MEAD.

the BRITISH phyfician looked upon profeffor BOERHAAVE's notions as chime-
rical, when he fought to cure the fmall
pox without fuppuration, by means of
a fpecific medicine extracted from *antimony* and *mercury* †. And the LEY-
DEN profeffor was perfuaded that the
afh colored ground liverwort was by
far, too highly extolled by Doctor
MEAD for the cure of the *hydrophobia*.
Thefe oppofite fentiments were candidly and amicably confidered, and did
not in the leaft decreafe the high opinion and confidence they had for each
other. In imitation of fuch venerable patterns, I have carefully expreffed
my thoughts as fully and clearly as I
could, without giving offence, or leffening in the leaft that refpectful tribute due to every perfon who exerts
his abilities for the common good of
mankind.—In this fection the external and internal ufe of *mercury*, for

* BOERHAAVE de materie medica, fect. 1392.
p. 256.

the

the prevention and cure of this difeafe are particularly confidered.

The fourth fection contains cafes and obfervations tending to illuftrate and confirm by facts, the fuccefs of the method which was purfued. Although the number be but fmall, there being only feven, yet from thefe may be drawn fufficient confirmation of the variety of the diftemper, according to the fex, conftitution of the patient, and feafon of the year. The firft two cafes are plainly acute. The three following are doubtful. The fixth of the putrid kind. And the feventh flow. Of thefe I am under the higheft obligations to Doctor HELE of SALISBURY, and to my very worthy friend CHARLES ALLIX, Efq; for their kind communications. And as in an enquiry of this nature, even few well attefted facts ferve greatly to afcertain the truth of an efficacious practice, fo trials made by different perfons, and fuch who are not of the profeffion, will corroborate a teftimo-

ny,

ny, and fatisfy thofe who may have but an unfavorable opinion of medicine and phyficians.

To every cafe I have fubjoined my remarks, and I flatter myfelf, that the freedom I have taken will not be difagreeable to the authors of them, efpecially to Doctor NUGENT, whofe ingenious Effay on the *hydrophobia*, and remarkable cafe of ELIZABETH BRYANT, I could not pafs over without paying it due regard.

It may be obferved, that in my remarks upon the cafe of FRANCIS RAY, I have taken no notice of Doctor JAMES's fever powder given by Mr. ALLIX, and left I fhould appear to be biaffed or prejudiced, I think it but fair to declare, that I am fully convinced Mr. ALLIX gave it to FRANCIS RAY with no other intention, than to quicken the operation of the fea water which he fent, and whofe purgative quality he feared might be leffened confiderably by being ftale.   Doctor JAMES feems in the

6   cafe

cafe of WILLIAM GOODACRE *, to at-
tribute the cure of that perfon in the
hydrophobia, to have been owing to
his powder; but it doth not appear that
this man had been bitten by a mad
dog, and moft probably the fymptoms
of the *hydrophobia* in the fmall-pox,
were no other than what are obferved
in acute fevers, efpecially of a putrid
nature, where the nerves of the *œfophagus* are particularly affected.   I do
not pretend to know, nor will I allow myfelf the liberty of guefling at the con-
tents of that fever powder, which I own
I never faw.   From the effects which
I have feen, it is a medicine of a powerful nature; it may undoubtedly have
been of fervice in the beginning of fevers, in diflodging the putrid *faburra*
from the firft paffages where it lodged,
and caufed the flame, but this I can
fafely add, from my own obfervation,
that the purging, vomiting, and profufe fweats which attend it's operation,

* JAMES's Differtation on fevers, p. 50.

a 2   cannot

cannot be safe in such a relaxed, low, and depressed state, wherein the *vis vitæ* is almost exhausted. In the recital of so many cases to recommend the sale of this powder, it were to be wished that in justice to mankind those also had been inserted wherein it had failed, as so many cautions to avoid the improper administration of it. A physician who has the welfare of his patient and reputation at heart, can never direct a medicine whose composition and ingredients he is a stranger to, let his desire of relieving his patient in the speediest manner be ever so laudable and just. And on the other hand, such physicians are rather to be commended than blamed for their tenderness and humanity, when after declining to prescribe this powder, they have generously attended their patients, to watch and guard them against the violent effects of so active a medicine which they have taken of their own accord, or by the persuasion of their zealous friends.

After

After all, Doctor JAMES who has alfo inferted WILLIAM GOODACRE's cafe
in his *treatife on canine madnefs*; *p.* 7,
8. " owns that he could not difcover
" the man had been bitten by a mad
" animal to occafion the *hydrophobia*,
" nor does he know in that cafe that
" his powders would have cured him."

Laftly, in the conclufion, after en-
quiring into the caufe of the general
alarm, fpread over the metropolis on
account of mad dogs, fome directions
are given for the treatment of the difeafe, occafioned by the bite of a mad
dog.

This is the fubftance of the Effay,
now offered to the public, and which
fhould have been publifh'd fome months
ago, when it was drawn up, had not
the advertifing of Doctor JAMES's *treatife on the canine madnefs* retarded it's
appearance, but on perufing that work
and finding nothing to prevent this
publication, I venture to fubmit my
thoughts on the fame fubject, to the

examina-

examination of every candid reader, whom I would firſt apprize, that I claim ſo little merit in this performance as truly to be able to ſay with the poet,

Vix ea noſtra voco.

for I have only illuſtrated and attempted to reconcile the various opinions of others, and to fix upon the moſt rational method of cure from a full conviction, that ſuch cure is in reality a practicable thing.

Let the reader then judge candidly of this performance, which if it prove the means of leſſening the general and too ſtrong rivetted apprehenſions of the diſeaſe, and alſo contributes to the prevention or cure of it, I ſhall think I have not miſ-ſpent my time, nor forfeited the good will and favor of my countrymen.

T H E

THE
CONTENTS.

INTRO-

INTRODUCTION.

SIR Thomas Browne †, in his enquiries into vulgar and common errors, among other caufes of decep-
tion, places credulity, authority, and
adherence to antiquity; and no doubt, as he
obferves, through the natural infirmity of human nature, through a fupinenefs and readi-
nefs to believe whatever is tranfmitted, by a
tradition feemingly authentic, and diftinguifhed
with authority, men are led implicitly to adopt
the opinions of their forefathers, to propagate
them with the fame confidence as if they had
been eye-witneffes of what they affert, and
thus hand down to pofterity the errors they
early imbibed, and never gave themfelves the
trouble of inquiring into. But although mankind is not quite free from thofe prejudices,
which are fo many obftructions to the ad-
vancement of every art and fcience, yet daily
experience teftifies, that in an enlightened age
popular notions are not fo univerfally adhered

† Sir Thomas Browne's Enquiries into received te-
nets, and prefumed truths, book i. chap. iv, v, vi, vii.

to, unlefs they be eftablifhed by repeated experiments, and matter of fact.

Indeed now-a-days, fome men run into another extreme, and from a predominant principle of vanity, reject, as fo many idle tales, or falfe conjectures, every thing, which doth not immediately ftrike them, not only withholding their affent, but even refufing to examine, into the truth of whatever is propofed to their confideration.   Thus it is hard to fay, which of the two, credulity, or fcepticifm, has proved the greater obftacle to the improvement of natural knowlege.   It is plain, that both have ended in a ftrong fpirit of enthufiafm, and that, in the art of medicine, as in other liberal arts, men through credulity, authority, adherence to antiquity, and alfo through fcepticifm, have been ftrangely mifled.   But the true Philofopher fteers a middle courfe, and avoids both thofe extremes; he refpects the authority of the ancients, without yielding his affent to what is either unnatural, or improbable; nor does he haftily condemn them, in favor of new difcoveries, unlefs thefe are confirmed by repeated experience.   On the other hand, he does not reject whatever is offered contrary to ancient authority, but candidly examines, what is propofed on both fides, and agrees to every new improvement, which bears the teft of repeated examination.

Had not this been the rule which feveral great men have obferved, the art of medicine

would,

would, at this time, have been as much a conjectural art, as in the time of CELSUS*. It's certainty, indeed, can never be expected to be absolute, while there are, and muft neceffarily be, fuch a variety of conftitutions, and of courfe fuch different degrees, as well as fpecies, of the fame diftemper.

It is therefore the Phyfician's province, to difcover the nature of the difeafe, the variety of its degrees, and appearance in different conftitutions and climates, and to regulate his practice accordingly.

But to this great end, he muft previoufly be acquainted with the conftruction of the human body, and the laws of the animal œconomy. It will not be fufficient alone to know the texture of the folids, without examining alfo the fluids. The knowlege of the circulation of the blood, which difcovery will ever be the greateft honor to our countryman Doctor HARVEY, can avail but little, if the conftituent parts of the blood are not examined, and, in the courfe of its circulation, the feveral fecretions are not traced, the recrements and excrements obferved, that by thefe inquiries the conftitution and ftrength of every perfon may be determined.

Thus, by joining to what the ancients have remarked on thefe fubjects, the improvements that have arifen from later experiments, the

* CELSUS De Medicina, in præfatione, p. 13—57.

great

great advantages proceeding from both will be happily united. The art of medicine will then appear, as Dr. BARKER fays †, to have a fettled rule of practice; and allowing for the difference of climate and conftitution, the precepts of the *ancients*, and directions of the *moderns*, will be eafily reconciled, according to their feveral notions of thofe difeafes which repeated experience had made familiar.

Whenever any acute difeafe hath alarmed mankind, by its rapid progrefs, or baneful deftruction, fo as to have produced the greateft fears on its appearance, and defpondency on its firft effects, men have embraced, with the utmoft eagernefs, whatever method of relief has been offered, in the hope of receiving a fpeedy and inftantaneous cure. This is remarkably the cafe with refpect to that diftemper, in particular, which is intended to be the fubject of the following Effay.

There is not a more dreadful difeafe incident to human nature than that which we are liable to from the bite of a mad dog. The fymptoms of it are terrible, the confequences are generally fatal, and the cure hitherto uncertain. The reflection on fuch an unhappy fituation, which inftantly occurs to a perfon bitten, difpofes him to hearken, with implicit fubmiffion, to the opinion and advice of every one in whom he has the leaft confidence: the

† BARKER's Effay on the agreement between ancient and modern phyficians, chap. i.

the * boasted remedies of the ancients, or empirical jumbles of later times, are applied in vain, the poison gains ground, and the patient, seeing himself disappointed, begins to doubt of the possibility of his being saved, and adds to the fury of the disease by his despondency and despair; till at last the aggravated symptoms relieve him from misery, by a welcome death, or which was the custom, not a century past, the unfortunate person was, contrary to all rules of humanity, deprived of life, by being smothered between two feather-beds †.

To prevent, therefore, all ill consequences arising from vulgar and common errors, the nature and effects of this poison, on the animal œconomy, the different methods of cure recommended in all times, and the few cures performed, are candidly to be examined, and mankind freed, if possible, from that most terrible reflection, that providence should have permitted the whole animal creation to be liable to so dreadful a disease, without pointing out, also, the means of cure.

That this distemper is not absolutely incurable, many instances plainly prove; and professor BOERHAAVE is of opinion, " That " from the examples already settled, and con- " firmed in the cases of other poisons, we

---

* BOERHAAVII Aphorismi, 1139, 1141.
† MEAD's Essays on poisons, p. 176.

" ought

" ought not to defpair of finding out the pro-
" per antidote for this alfo *."

In the courfe of this Effay I fhall endeavor
to prove, that this difeafe is of a complicated
kind, having different appearances according
to the age, ftrength, conftitution, fex, and
manner of life of the perfon bitten, tempe-
rature of the climate he inhabits, and the feafon of the year in which the accident happens; and alfo, that as circumftances of this
fort are found to vary in particular cafes, the
method of treatment is to be varied likewife.

---

* Nec defperandum tamen, ob exempla, jam in aliis
venenis conftantia, de inveniendo hujus fingularis veneni
antidoto fingulari. BOERHAAVII Aphorifmus, 1146.
VAN SWIETEN Commentar. in BOERHAAVII Aphorifmos,
tom. iii. p. 579.

SECTION I.

Of the Bite of a Mad Dog.

BEfore I proceed to give an account of the fymptoms occafioned by the bite of a mad dog, it may not be improper to obferve,

Firſt, That wounds made by the bite of a perfon, in the height of anger, of enraged animals, or wild beaſts, are always attended with fevere accidents: thefe are owing, as CELSUS declares *, very properly, not to any particular poifon in the animal, but to the violent laceration and compreſſion of the muſcles, nerves, tendons, veſſels, ligaments, and bones; particularly in the bite of a large dog, of an horfe, a wolf, a bear, or any fuch fized creature whofe tufks and teeth either fqueeze and bruife the parts they lay hold of, with fo much force, as to make a deep wound, or tear away with exquifite pain, whenever their teeth have not entered fo deeply. The fymptoms arifing from thefe bites, are, to the full, as violent as thofe which attend lacerated wounds

---

* CELSUS, lib. v. cap. 27.
  HEISTERI Chirurgia, part. i. lib. i. cap. xvi. p. 160.

occa-

occafioned by any blunt-pointed or rough in-
ftrument whatever; the lofs of fubftance, and
the parts affected, determining the violence of
the fymptoms, and the length of time requifite for obtaining a cure, according to the degree ot fuppuration, and conftitution of the
patient.

Secondly, Such is the fermentation raifed
in the blood, by the paffion of anger, that the
momentum of the circulation is greatly increafed, and the fecretion of the *faliva* forced
out, in a larger quantity, by the frequent pul-
fation and compreffion of the blood-veffels.
Such perfons, or creatures, who are lefs liable
to fweat, have generally a more copious difcharge of urine; but in a violent fit of anger,
the urinary fecretion is fufpended, and they
throw out large quantities of *faliva*, which
appears the more frothy, the more the perfon
or animal is enraged, according to the velocity of the circulation of the blood, which is
fometimes increafed to fuch a degree, as to
produce an high fever, attended with *delirium*
and convulfions, and which, in fome inftances,
brings on an apoplexy, and death.

Thirdly, That the *faliva* of a man, an
horfe, a monkey, and even of a dog, is not
poifonous in a found ftate, nor even when
they are provoked to anger, common experience daily proves. The *faliva* is a thin,
tranfparent humor, which, heated on the fire,
doth not thicken, is free from tafte or fmell,

froths

froths when ſtrongly ſhaken, and is a glandular juice ſeparated from pure arterial blood, and conſiſting of water, ſpirit, oil, and ſome ſalt *. Now I ſhall only aſk, Whether it is not univerſally admitted, that medicinally the *ſaliva*, both of man and animals, have been recommended externally as detergents, and dryers? Is it not known that many perſons have found benefit from training up young dogs daily to lick foul ulcers, which no ointment could cleanſe ſo well? And Lord Bacon † has long ſince taken notice of it as a common obſervation, That dogs are almoſt the only beaſts which delight in fetid odors; whence their readineſs to lick their own, and other ſores, may be accounted for: and there never was known a ſingle inſtance in which the *ſaliva* of a young dog, although it has effectually acted as the moſt powerful deterſive on ulcers, and has been received on thoſe ulcers, when bleeding, hath produced the leaſt ſigns of madneſs, or *hydrophobia*,—merely becauſe the dog was in a ſound ſtate.

No other ſymptoms, therefore, will ariſe after the bite of an angered perſon, or an enraged animal, ſuch as an horſe, a monkey, or a dog, than will appear from a lacerated and contuſed wound violently compreſſed and torn.

* Boerhavii Inſtitutiones Medicæ, v. 66.
† Bacon's Sylva Sylvarum, cent. ix. v. 835. Epiſtle on fetid and fragrant odors.

I come

I come now to confider what may be the caufe of madnefs in dogs and other animals, and to defcribe the fymptoms which attend the bite of thofe animals when mad.

PALMARIUS *, a difciple of FERNELIUS, who gives a circumftantial account of this madnefs, defcribes it to be a rage which feizes dogs at any time of the year, but chiefly during that part of the fummer called the dog-days; that they communicate this madnefs by contact, both to man and beaft. Whenever a dog, an animal eafily provoked to anger, of a natural propenfity to become furious, is kept from drink, either during the exceffive heat of the fummer, or the fharp cold in the winter †, his bile acquires fuch an extraordinary degree of acrimony, that he grows mad: but if thefe contrary difpofitions of the atmofphere affect his blood and humours in fuch a manner that he become furious, it often alfo happens, that, through long fafting, being filled with falt meats or falt drink, or through want of drink after long and laborious exercife, a dog runs mad: and, particularly, if a dog has been bitten by one mad, or hath eaten of the flefh of any animal dead of madnefs, or of the plague, or of any putrid difeafe, killed by lightning, or by poifon,

---

* JULIUS PALMARIUS Conftantius De morbis contagiofis.

† DIOSCORIDES De Theriaca, cap. i. Signa rabiofi canis, eorumque qui ab eo demorfi fuerunt.

or

or hath drank of ftinking and corrupted waters, or eaten of high-feafoned acrid food, or
hath worms;—in any one of thefe cafes he is
liable to go mad.   Therefore in fuch countries where the change of air is fudden or extreme, fometimes violently hot, at other times
intenfely cold, this difeafe, in proportion, is
more common ‖.

An inftance of the fudden effect of cold on
a dog, I fhall here relate.   In the month of
February 1744, on a clear frofty morning, a
perfon of my acquaintance going from his
houfe in *Dean-ftreet,* near *Soho-Square*, to
Mary la bonne, took out with him a fmall
dog, of a fpurious breed, partly fpaniel, and
partly harlequin, which had been kept within
doors all the preceding part of the winter.
The little creature was much delighted with
his liberty, and running to and fro', when
near *Cavendifh-Square*, his mafter faw him
reel, and ftagger; upon which, he took the
dog up into his arms, and was rubbing his
legs, on the fide he thought was benumbed
with the cold, when, on a fudden, the dog
was obferved to froth confiderably at the
mouth, his eyes were red like fire, and immediately, from being a timorous and fond
animal, he began to fnap at his mafter, and
attempted, feveral times, to bite him.—On

‖ Boerhaavii Aphorifmus, 1134. Van Swieten
Comment. tom. iii. p. 539. Mead's Effays on poifons,
p. 137.

this,

this, convinced of the danger he was in, the gentleman threw him out of his arms, and the dog ran fwiftly down the next ftreet, where he was purfued into a meufe. He then endeavored to bite a large dog, which avoided him, and afterwards ran at fome coach-horfes which the farrier was fhoeing; but upon his mafter's calling out to the man, the dog was prevented from doing any mifchief, by a fortunate ftroke of the farrier's hammer, which at once put the poor animal alfo out of pain.

Such is the pernicious virulence of the *faliva* thrown out by a mad dog, that all kinds of animals whatfoever, fuch as monkeys, fwine, cats, oxen, horfes, fheep, mules, foxes, wolves, and others, are not only liable to grow mad, upon being bitten; but alfo have, without any bite, been feized with the *hydrophobia* upon the fole contact and admiffion of a mad dog's *faliva,* And PALMA-RIUS † relates an inftance of a countryman, who raving mad of this difeafe, and being informed he had not long to live, defired, in an intermiffion of his fits, that he might take his laft farewel of his children, which the people who kept him tied down having confented to, he kiffed them, and then was fuffocated. However, on the feventh day the children were feized with the fame illnefs, and died in the fame cruel agonies and pains. He alfo

† PALMARIUS loc. cit.

has

has feen cattle killed by eating ftraw on which the flabber of mad animals had been left.

* Coelius Aurelianus records a quicker progrefs of the infected *faliva*. He fays, that a certain botcher-woman having taken a coat to mend, which had been torn by a mad dog, having drawn the threads through her lips to make them ftick together, and having moiftened the feams with her tongue, that her needle might pafs through the eafier, ran mad the third day.

Notwithftanding Galen afferts ||, that dogs are the only animals which become mad without being bitten, or the leaft communication; many of the abovementioned creatures grow furious without any previous infection, but none fo frequently as dogs, foxes, and wolves †. Palmarius ‡ has feen twenty wolves, driven mad through hunger, fally out of a foreft, and feize every living creature that came in their way, none of which efcaped who were bitten.

---

* Sartrix etiam quædam quum chlamydem fciffam rabidis morfibus, farciendam fumeret, atque ore ftamina componeret, & lingua pannorum futuras lamberet, affuendo quo tranfitum acus faceret faciliorem, tertia die in *rabiem* veniffe memoratur. Coelius Aurelianus De morbis acutis, lib. iii. cap. ix.

|| Galenus, lib. vi. De loc. affect.

† Boerhavii Aphorifmi, 1132, 1133.

‡ Palmarius, loc. cit.

Doctor Lister*, and Doctor Mead †, affign the true caufe of the violent fermentation, raifed in the blood of dogs either through heat or cold, by obferving, " That no dog " ever fweats; and that as next to the miliary " glands in the human body, the falival glands " are the moft conftant and eafy emuncto- " ries, through which the faline and active " particles of the blood are difcharged, more " fpittle is feparated in a dog, when mad, " than at any other time, and that very " frothly, or impregnated with hot fubtil " parts."

Now whenever this difcharge is obftructed, by too great a vifcidity of the blood, from an increafed circulation and want of dilution, the confequence of long thirft; then the faline particles grow more acrid, and the abforbed bilious falts particularly acquire fuch acrimony, as to produce a high fever and *delirium*, by irritating the nerves, difturbing the fecretion and courfe of the nervous fluid, and throwing all the laws of the animal œconomy into confufion, exciting fuch different and various fymptoms, in perfons of different fexes, and conftitutions, according as Doctor Mead rightly fays, to the paffions of the mind they are moft inclined to. And in this morbid ftate of a dog's *faliva* the fymptoms will be

* Lister, Exercitatio iii², p. 133.
† Mead, Effay on poifons, p. 138.

more

more aggravated, than thofe which attend the bite of an angered animal that is found, and the patient will be in greater danger. Or whenever the blood and juices of a dog, cat, wolf, or fox, fhall be fo vitiated as to become putrid, by either of the caufes already recited, then will a perfon, bitten by fuch animal, be expofed to all the fatal accidents which the admiffion of fuch a putrid, high fermenting *faliva* muft naturally produce, by mixing with the blood and humors, particularly the nervous fluid, which is remarkably affected in putrid difeafes of all kinds, but efpecially in peftilential and bilious fevers, wherein the acrimonious falts of the putrid bile abforbed into the blood, and alfo the diffolved ftate of the blood, which foon follows, vitiate the nervous fluid, at the fame time that the coats of the nerves are both irritated and relaxed. Hence thofe irregular fpafms, and involuntary contractions, all over the body, which bring on a tenfion, ftronger convulfions, and at length, by drying up the nerves, and deftroying the fluid commonly called the animal fpirits, put an end to the motion of the neceffary fprings of life.

This difeafe, therefore, is of a different nature, and even more or lefs complicated, according to the feafon of the year, and to the ftate of the juices belonging to the mad animal, whether found or morbid. Obftruction of perfpiration will, in winter, produce fever,

deli-

delirium and phrenzy, or madnefs; long fafting, thirft, after violent exercife, falted, fpiced,
and all acrid meats: likewife * worms bred
in the ftomach, inteftines, and at the root of
the nofe, will have the fame bad effects of producing madnefs, and the active particles of the
dog, cat, wolf, or fox's *faliva*, rendered more
fubtil by the increafed momentum of the
blood, will be capable of infecting man or any
animal that they fhall bite with the fame fer-
mentating principles, and of bringing on the
fame fatal fymptoms.

In fummer, the humors of the body affected by tainted air, food, or by ftagnating and
corrupted waters filled with innumerable infects, both living and dead, are fubject to a
putridity, which is afterwards increafed by the
velocity of the blood rarefied particularly in the
fummer, and even in autumn, through the
heat of the feafon. In man, this produces an

---

* Some authors have been fond of the notion, that not
only the *hydrophobia*, but the fmall-pox, the *Lues Venerea*
all cutaneous eruptions, and many other diforders are produced by worms, generated in the feveral humours of the
body. That worms are admitted and multiplied in the
firft paffages, and under the integuments both of man and
beaft, and occafion various complaints, common experience daily fhows. But as profeffor ASTRUC has refuted,
the exiftence of worms in venereal cafes, I fhall refer the
reader to his opinion †, which will hold good in ahe examination of the vitiated *faliva* of a mad dog, in which no
one as yet proved the appearance of any fuch vermin.

† ASTRUC de morbis venereis, tom. i. lib. ii. c. ii. p. 127, & feq. tom.
ii. p. 1067.

acute

acute, or a bilious fever, which deprives the
folids of their contractile force, deftroys the
animal fpirits, inflames the membranes of the
brain, brings on a *delirium*; and either kills
the perfon by convulfions, or by changing the
whole mafs of blood into *pus*, expofes the patient either to critical tumors, difcharges of
matter, a *marafmus*, or to fome chronical difeafe, unlefs timely prevented. In the brute
creation, the progrefs would be the fame, were
they not deftroyed as foon as the fever appears, efpecially if attended with a phrenzy; for no fooner doth the *delirium* feize them,
than that fatal effect of their biting comes on,
and the blood then being in its higheft degree
of fermentation, has the more power to infect
other bodies, and raife the fame furious fymptoms in them.

It appears therefore, that in different feafons of the year, there is a latent difpofition
in the fluids of dogs towards acrimony and putridity, which according to the various effects
of thofe feafons manifefts itfelf; and from an
innocent fecretion, turns the *faliva* of a dog
to a moft dangerous poifon.

Here it may not be improper to defcribe the
figns of the feveral degrees of madnefs in dogs *.

The

---

* In Sir Theodore Mayern's account, publifhed
from his papers, by Sir Theodore de Vaux, there are
reckoned up no lefs than feven diftinct forts of madnefs or
difeafes, peculiar to dogs. 1. The *hot madnefs*. 2. The

C

running

The madnefs, which through cold, feizes thefe animals like a phrenzy in winter, comes on fo fuddenly, as to afford no time for obfervation or caution, and many inftances might be produced of houfe-dogs or others, biting their mafters and keepers, without the leaft previous notice ; and of the fame furious effects being raifed in the perfon bitten, by means of the acrimonious falts contained in the blood of the animal, and now let loofe and difcharged in its *faliva*.

In all feafons of the year, but particularly in fummer and autumn, the madnefs arifing from a putrid ftate of the blood doth not come on fo fuddenly : there are manifeft figns of the animal being ill ; the progrefs of the difeafe is gradual ; and either quicker or flower, according to the elafticity and refiftance of the folids, and the degree of putrefcence, and acrimony of the falts circulating in the fluids.

The figns of a dog going to run mad, are thefe. He is firft feized with a fhaking and trembling, then grows thin, feems dejected, hides himfelf, refufes to eat or drink, hangs down his ears and tail, fneaks away growling, howls at times in a particular manner, flies

running madnefs. 3. *La rage mue*, or the *fullen madnefs*. 4. The *falling madnefs*, or *epilepfy*. 5. The *blafting* or *withering*. 6. The *fleepy madnefs* owing to worms. 7. The *rheumatic* difeafe. Of thefe he fays, the two firft are to be catched by the breath of dogs, and are incurable ; the five laft contagious, but curable. Philofophical Tranfactions, N°. 191.

upon

upon ftrangers, and carries his head as if he were fleepy. His eyes are watery, his noftrils drawn clofe, and difcharging *mucus*, his mouth open, and running with his tongue dry, and of a bilious color.

In the fecond degree of madnefs, which is by far the moft dangerous; a dog forgets his mafter, lay's hold without diftinction, of every perfon or animal who comes in his way, and without barking, bites and tears whatever he feizes. He now cannot fwallow, and turns away at the fight of water. He opens his mouth wide, pants for breath, froths confiderably, hangs his tongue quite out, which now turns of a livid color. His eyes are inflamed, and of a fiery red. He at times runs on furioufly, at other times ftands or lies down as if ftupid, or half afleep; particularly during the remiffion of the fever, which conftantly attends thefe fymptoms, and whofe paroxyfms, and exacerbations are regular*. In this condition, all other dogs fhun him, and if they cannot well avoid him, they yield, and endeavor to footh him.

There are feveral methods recommended by PALMARIUS and others, to difcover whether a dog is mad that has bit a perfon, and has either made his efcape, or been killed before the figns of madnefs could be obferved, Firft, to apply a pultice of bruifed walnuts to the

---

* PALMARIUS loc. cit.

wound

wound, and let it lie on the whole night, and
then give it to chicken for food, and if the dog
which has efcaped is mad, the chicken will
die in a day or two.   Secondly, to fop up the
blood running from the wound with a piece
of crumb of bread, and offer it to dogs to eat,
which they will refufe, if the dog was mad;
or to feed fowls with the fame fop, which will
kill them in twenty-four hours, if the dog was
in that dangerous ftate.   Another method advifed, where the dog has been killed, is to rub
his mouth, jaws and nofe with a piece of bread,
fo as to moiften it with the *faliva*, and in the
fame manner offer it to dogs, or to feed fowls
with the fame intention.

Some perfons affirm, that fuch dogs as have
been wormed, never bite others, although they
run mad either fpontaneoufly, or after being
bitten by a mad dog, but no reliance is to be
made upon fuch an affurance; fince it is plain,
that the danger of being infected is entirely owing to the admiffion of the *faliva*, which may
have the fame bad effect, being licked up by o-
ther dogs, or received into any wound; although
perhaps the *virus* may not be fo fpeedy in its progrefs, as when immediately conveyed by the
bite of the infected animal.   The extraction
therefore of part of the *frænum* of the tongue,
can be of no real ufe to prevent this calamity.

It is to be obferved, that the *faliva* of a
mad dog, cat, or other animal has no bad effect on the fkin, any more than the venereal,
the

the leprous, or any other *virus* *, provided the
ſkin be whole, and that the part on which the
ſaliva has fixed be immediately cleanſed and
well waſhed †.

· But whenever the *ſaliva* of a mad dog is received into a wound, it takes the ſame courſe
as the variolous matter, or the venereal taint;
indeed in general, it is quicker in its progreſs,
unleſs in ſome particular conſtitutions, wherein
it has been known to lie dormant months and
years ‖. But the *ſaliva* of a viper, a rattle-
ſnake, or a *tarantula* is quickeſt of all in its
effects, which however vary, as to the time
of their appearance in different conſtitutions;
and as REDI remarks, the *ſaliva* of the viper
frequently produces the moſt cruel and violent
ſymptoms, bringing the creature bitten to the
very brink of death, and yet the animal is not
deſtroyed, but is cured without help or medicine, and by the ſole power of nature ‡.

Children and young people are affected in
a ſtronger manner, and ſooner than perſons
more advanced in years §; owing no doubt to
the different degree of velocity in the circulation of their blood. But no caution is

---

* STALPART VANDER WIELEN, Obſervat. rarior cen-
tur. i. p. 413.

† Du CHOISEL's method of treating perſons bit by mad
animals, p. 20.

‖ FREIND, Hiſtoria Medicinæ, 4to, p. 208. MEAD's
Eſſays on poiſons.

‡ REDI Experimenta Naturalia, p. 262.

§ Du CHOISEL's method, p. 18.

 to

to be omitted, for although Monf. SAU-
VAGES * fays, that men are more liable to the
moft violent effects of this poifonous *faliva* than
women; yet BARON VAN SWIETEN † obferves
thereupon, that men, by fweating through hard
labor, may have difcharged the venomous
virus, while a perfon of a more tender, delicate,
and cooler conftitution, may feel the effects later,
and die with more eafe. An inftance which
I faw, will alfo comparatively fhew the various
effects of the *faliva* of a mad dog, on different
fpecies and conftitutions of the fame animal.

In *June* 1758, a mad dog ran into the court-
yard belonging to the Rev. Doctor FAVELL,
of *Witton*, in the county of *Huntingdon*: He
bit a pointer in the heels, fought and tore two
fpaniel bitches, who then were fuckling their
puppies, a fpaniel dog, and a greyhound bitch;
after which he ran into the town, bit other
dogs and a child. Three days after, near the
full moon, the two bitches fickned, their milk
dried up, they had not the *hydrophobia*, but
died, as it were fuffocated on the fifth day,
without violent figns of madnefs, or any power of running or biting; but delirious and conftantly barking and howling in a particular
hoarfe manner. On the feventh, the pointer
grew dull, then furious, and was fhot. The
greyhound continued well, till the next full

* SAUVAGES differtation fur la nature, & caufe de la rage,
p. 7. Ann. 1748.
† VAN SWIETEN Comment. tom. iii. p. 549.

moon,

.moon, when she became mopish, avoided
company, and snarled at those she was generally fond of; upon which the symptoms
increasing, she was strangled. The other
dogs bitten in the town as well as the child,
were in no sort affected. This verifies the
opinions of all authors who have written on
this subject, that the same vitiated *saliva* may
have various effects according to the different
constitutions of the animal or person bitten.

* The general opinion of the most celebrated authors and practitioners, is, that the
poisonous *saliva* of a mad dog insinuates itself
into the wound made by the bite †, from
whence it is absorbed in like manner with the
variolous matter in the practice of inoculation,
or like the venereal *virus,* and circulates with
the blood; which by degrees it taints and affects the several humors, as also the nervous
fluid, called the animal spirits; and by stimulating, causes frequent spasmodic contractions
of the nerves,

Some account for the different progress of
this *saliva* in like manner with the venereal
virus, which according to professor BOER-
HAAVE and others, being lodged in the *cellular
membrane* and there sheathing itself in the oily

---

* PALMARIUS, De morsu canis rabidi, chap. i.
    BOERHAAVII Prælectiones Academicæ, de morbis
nervorum, tom. i. p. 214.
    MEAD's Essays on poisons. Introduct. p. 30, & seq.
† SAUVAGES dissertation sur la rage, p. 45.
    VAN SWIETEN Comment. tom. iii. p. 551.

subfubftance contained in the cells of the *membrana adipofa* lays dormant therein, until it be abforbed by the *lymphatics* and conveyed into the blood veffels, wherein it circulates with the blood, and mixing with it fooner or later, unfolds its active principles according as they have been more or lefs fheathed. This makes no doubt, the wide difference between the flow advances of thefe acrimonious falts in perfons of a lax or leucophlegmatic habit of body, or particularly when received into the fatty fubftance contained in the *cellular membrane*, and their quick progrefs when inftilled directly into the blood, which can feldom happen without wounding at the fame time the nerve which accompanies the blood-veffel; and thereby caufing thofe fpafmodic contractions and painful pulfations, which the known irritability of thofe parts will be liable to.

Others, however, will not allow that this poifonous *faliva* is conveyed by the blood, but account for all its effects from its *ftimulus* on the nerves, which are thrown into fpafms, convulfions, ftrictures, and involuntary contractions.

DOCTOR NUGENT adopts another fyftem. He feems, in his ingenious effay, p. 133—139. to acquiefce in the exiftence of a nervous fluid, commonly called the animal fpirits, but will not allow that they are tainted by the *faliva* of a mad dog, or that the feveral fymptoms are produced by their means: nay, he doubts, p. 147. whether, " although undoubtedly

" edly poifoned liquors get into the circula-
" tion, it is not probable that they carry none
" of their malignity with them, but leave it
" all among the fibres of the part they firft
" infect." And throughout the whole effay,
he endeavors to account for all the fymptoms
arifing from the bite of a mad dog, by the ac-
tion of the *virus* on the nervous fibres, whofe
vibrations and ofcillatory motions are firft by
the nibbling poifon thrown into *fpafmuli*, which
being repeated, are progreffively continued
from one nerve to another, till they are put into violent contractions and affect fome or other
of the *vifcera*.

It is not my defign, by any means, to enter
into a fruitlefs controverfy. The opinions of
PALMARIUS, profeffor BOERHAAVE, and doctor MEAD, are fufficient authorities for me;
and experience juftifies their affertion, that
the nervous fluid, whatever it may be, is generally tainted in the fever raifed by the bite of
a mad dog. It would be endlefs to quote all
they have faid; I fhall therefore only refer the
reader to profeffor BOERHAAVE's, and doctor
MEAD's thoughts, concerning the nervous
fluid or animal fpirits *. And with regard to
the effects of the bite of a viper, or the puncture of a nerve or tendon, they may vary greatly

---

* BOERHAAVII Aphorifmi & prælectiones academicæ
de morbis nervorum.
    MEAD, Effay on poifons, loc. cit.

in their confequences *; as poffibly the firft
may be deftitute of putridity, and yet have a
fufficient acrimony to throw the whole nervous fyftem into the fame fatal convulfions as
the puncture of a confiderable nerve, or tendon commonly doth.   But putrid difeafes in
general, and particularly thofe of the moft active kind, as the plague, the fmall-pox, and
Lues Venerea, are known to diffufe themfelves
all over the human body, and to affect diftinct
emunctories according to the different fhape,
figure and fize of their acrimonious falts. Thus
the peftilential matter affects the larger glands,
as the *parotid*, the *axillary*, and *inguinal*; the
fmall-pox, thofe of the fkin ; and the *Lues Venerea*, the tefticles, the *inguinal*, and *falival*
glands.

The putrid *faliva* of a mad dog has been
compared long ago to the venereal *virus*, in
its manner of being communicated and in its
progrefs, by ALEXANDER MASSARIAS †, profeffor of PADUA, as profeffor ASTRUC records.

The more the falts in thefe putrid difeafes
are exalted and volatilized, the more violent
is their effect on the nervous fyftem, and the
fooner is the nervous fluid tainted.

But to proceed to the fymptoms incident
upon the bite of a mad dog.   I have already

* Venenum peftilens, variolofum, rabiofum, alio modo communicatur, quam viperinum.   BOERHAAVII prælectiones academicæ de morbis nervorum, p. 214.

† ASTRUC de morbis venereis, p. 842.

men-

mentioned, that the pain and cure of the wound depended on the texture of the parts bitten; the same may be said of the bite of a mad animal as of an angered one; for the bites of mad dogs have been commonly found to heal without difficulty; indeed in some habits of body they scab over, and do not heal so firmly.

The firft effects of a poifonous *faliva*, appear rarely before the third day; fometimes not till the thirtieth or fortieth, and fome inftances are related of the poifon laying dormant two or three years; nay longer, and then breaking out *. It generally fhows itfelf at the full, or new moon †, when a fharp pricking pain is felt in the part where the bite was given, although the wound fhall have been healed fome time. Unlefs fome nervous or tendinous part be bitten, the pain at firft is not very violent, it foon however afcends, and fpreads itfelf all over the mufcles of that limb, caufing a wearinefs; then darts up towards the throat and heart, and occafions a weight on the *præcordia*, and a great oppreffion, a continual inquietude attended with fighings and fobbings, a dullnefs and love of folitude. The perfon's mind begins now to be affected, he grows peevifh and angry, and in his fleep he is difturbed, reftlefs, and frequently awakened by frightful dreams. In the fecond ftage of this difeafe

* ETMULLERI opera, tom. i. p. 504.
† MEAD's Effay on poifons, p. 152, 153.

all

all the above fymptoms increafe; then come
on flufhing heats, a burning heat at the pit of
the ftomach, *naufea*, vomiting of dark and vif-
cid matter, particularly a deep colored and
porraceous bile; a fever attended with horrors, tremblings, *fubfultus tendinum*, and convulfions.   A great thirft, drynefs of the throat,
hoarfnefs, difficulty of fwallowing liquids, but
a poffibility of admitting folids, a copious difcharge of the *faliva* like froth, which the patient avoids fwallowing *, a coftivenefs, pria-
pifms, or *furor uterinus* and *delirium*.

In the laft ftage, the patient is in the greateft fury; his madnefs increafes with every ex-
acerbation, and the remiffions are attended
with a cold fweat, as the pulfe and fever fail:
yet in the whole courfe of his fury he continues in his fenfes, and is fo far from being
mifchievous or attempting to bite, that he is
afraid of doing harm, and cautions the by
ftanders, left he fhould lofe his fenfes and prove
hurtful to them †.

His

---

* Lister exercitationes medicinales, exercit. iii². p.
114—117.

† Authors do not entirely agree in this point; but as the
generality are of opinion, that the unhappy perfons labor-
ing under this difeafe are not mifchievous even in very hot
climates, I think proper to quote their feveral fentiments,
that through fear of accidents fuch patients may not be de-
ferted, want proper affiftance, nor be put to a violent death,
which is no lefs than murder, if the cruel cuftom of fuffo-
cating them fhould ftill prevail in any civilized country, and
for which there can be no warrantable plea, fince inftances
are

His appearance now grows shocking to behold. His eyes are inflamed, staring, and wild; the tears flow involuntarily, his nostrils are spread, his mouth open, his tongue hanging out, rough and black; his voice extremely hoarse, his thirst intolerable, terrified at the sight of any liquid, particularly of water, and indeed of any shining or pellucid object; as any thing white, a looking-glass, &c. He froths at the mouth, endeavors to spit at the by-standers. Such is the sensibility of the nerves, that a glaring light, the least noise, or the smallest breeze of cool air, throws the patient into horrors, spasms, and convulsions. The last signs are, an extension and rigidity

are produced of persons being cured who had the *hydrophobia* strongly upon them.

Quibus addo, quod equidem neminem hactenus vel audiverim latrare vel viderim mordere. TULPII Obferv. Medic. lib. i. cap. xx.

Doctor MEAD says, that sometimes in their rage and fury they attempt doing all possible mischief to their most beloved friends and relations, but most commonly are melancholy, resigning themselves to death. Essay on poisons, p. 133.

Doctor DESAULT declares, that of all the persons whom he has seen seized with this madness, and that have even died raving, not one ever attempted to bite; nor did any counterfeit the actions or noise of animals, which had bit them. Dissertation sur la Rage, p. 322.

Monsieur DU CHOISEL saw only one instance of a young man who bit two women in the heighth of the fury. Method. p. 21. May not the heat of the climate, and constitution of the Indian, have produced this unusual effect? However, it is best to be upon one's guard in such cases.

of

of all the nerves *, a total inability of fwallowing liquids, a dread not only at the fight,
but even at the mention of them, a *vertigo*,
general convulfions, and death; which, from
the time this fatal difeafe is manifeft, happens
moftly on the third day, although it feldom ex-
ceeds the fourth.

In fuch bodies as have been opened after
this difeafe, it has appeared, that all the or-
gans of deglutition are inflamed, that the ftomach was filled with flimy and vifcous matter, mixed with bile of a dark and porraceous
color; that the gall-bladder was full of deep
green-colored bile, the *pericardium* generally quite dry, the lungs greatly diftended
with blood, the heart, and alfo the arteries,
full of a thin fluid blood, which doth not coa-
gulate in the air; the veins empty, and all the
membranes of the brain, *cerebellum*, *medulla
fpinalis*, and *vifcera*, dry.

From the above-mentioned view of the
bodies, and a confideration of the fymptoms
of this difeafe, doth it not appear, very plainly,
that the putrid fermentative *faliva* of a mad
dog circulates along with the blood †, acts as a
powerful *ftimulus* on the nerves and nervous
coats of the arteries, renders the faline particles of the blood and humors more active
and acrid, keeps the blood in a diffolved ftate,

---

* *Hydrophobia* homini evenit cum diftenfione nervorum.
LISTER Exercit. iiiª.

† MEAD's Effay on poifons, p. 140.

is

is difcharged by the falival glands down the *œfophagus* into the ftomach, caufing, in its courfe, a drynefs, tenfion, pain, and inflammation, and throwing all the nerves, by its irritation, into fpafms and contractions, which produce the difficulty of breathing, and of fwallowing liquids ? That in a ftate of putridity the nervous power being deftroyed, the heart and arteries can no longer contract, and therefore are found full of blood ; and that the acrimony of the bile, being increafed by long fafting, and want of dilution *, adds to the violent effects on the firft paffages, and helps alfo to affect the brain, and, confequently, the whole nervous fyftem ?

* Mr. HOLLWELL, in his Narrative of the deplorable death of the gentlemen fuffocated at CALCUTTA, defcribes very ftrongly the terrible effects arifing from the abforption of the bile into the blood ; the circulation of which was raifed by the tumultuous paffions of the mind, rage and defpair, and the bilious falts being highly volatilized for want of air to breathe, and of liquids to dilute during the profufe fweats of the confined perfons, brought on a *delirium*, lofs of ftrength, and, to fuch as furvived, putrid fevers.

SECTION

SECTION II.

Of the Hydrophobia.

COELIUS AURELIANUS, a phyfician of the methodic fect, who lived, as Monfieur LE CLERC records * from REINESIUS, about the fifth century of the Chriftian æra, is the firft author who has written largely of the *hydrophobia*, and defcribed all the fymptoms of it, with any tolerable exactnefs. In his time it was matter of great difpute among the phyficians, whether the *hydrophobia* was known to the ancients, or was a new difeafe? The reafons alledged on both fides, may be feen at length in his treatife *De Morbis acutis* †. He is clear in his opinion in favor of the ancients; intimating, that although HIPPOCRATES does not particularly treat of this difeafe, yet he may be fuppofed to have alluded to it in the following fentences ‖.

Οἱ φρενιτικοὶ ϐραχυποῖαι, ψοφᵤ, καϑαπῖόμενοι, τρομώδεες.

* LE CLERC Hiftoire de la Medecine, p. 556.
† COELIUS AURELIANUS, lib. iii. cap. xv.
‖ HIPPOCRATES a FOESIO, lib. i. Prædict. p. 68. & coacarum prænotionum.
VAN SWIETEN Commentar. tom. iii. p. 536.

Phre-

Phrenitici parùm bibunt, ex levibus ſtrepitibus facilè irritantur, ac percelluntur, tremuli ſunt.

Οἱ φρενίλιχοὶ Ϛραχυπόλαι ψοφȣ, καϑαπλομενοὶ τρομώδεες, ἤ σπασμώδεες.

Phrenitici parùm bibunt, ex levibus ſtrepitibus facilè irritantur, tremuli ſunt, aut convulſionibus tentantur.

Perſons in a phrenzy drink very little, are diſturbed and frightned, tremble on the leaſt noiſe, or are ſeized with convulſions.

ARETÆUS *, in treating of the cure for phrenitics, mentions the very ſame.

† The methodics ranked all diſeaſes under two claſſes; thoſe which were cauſed by ſtricture, or tenſion, and thoſe cauſed by relaxation. COELIUS AURELIANUS places the *hydrophobia* among the diſeaſes cauſed by ſtricture, or tenſion ; and ſays, " That it is poſ-
" ſible for the ſame paſſion to be produced in
" bodies, without any manifeſt cauſe, when-
" ever a ſtricture is ſpontaneouſly occaſioned,
" like that which ariſeth from poiſon ‖."

* ARETÆUS De Morbis acutis, edit. BOERHAAVII, lib. i. p. 72. C. Ibid. p. 77. B.

† LE CLERC Hiſtoire de la Medecine.

‖ Eſt præterea poſſibile ſine manifeſta cauſa, hanc paſſionem corporibus innaſci, cum talis fuerit ſtrictio, ſpontè generata qualis a veneno. COELIUS AURELIANUS, lib. iii. cap. ix.

D There

There is a great difference to be made between the difficulty of fwallowing ‡ which
arifes from a relaxation, and that which is
known to attend the *hydrophobia.* In para-
lytic diforders frequently attending upon old
age, and in fome forts of *anginæ,* neither folids nor liquids can be allowed to pafs; and
the very attempt has endangered the patient,
who has been almoft fuffocated. But to this
* difficulty of fwallowing, in the *hydrophobia,*
a real † dread of water fucceeds, particularly
in thofe conftitutions, and in that advanced
ftate of the difeafe, when the ftricture or tenfion is fo great, the acrimony fo confiderable,
the inflammation fo high, the fever fo ftrong
in its exacerbations, and the irregular fpafms
of the nerves fo far increafed from partial
contractions to general convulfions, that the
fear of fuffocation is become continual; in
which cafe alfo it appears plainly, that the patient's mind is as much affected as the body.

‖ Coelius Aurelianus has written a
whole chapter to prove, that the *hydrophobia*
                                                    is

---

‡ Medical Effays, vol. i. art. xxvii. - Dr. Gilbert
Waugh's account of Hart's daughter.

* Δυσκαταπoσις.

† Ὑδροφοβία.

‖ Coelius Aurelianus, lib. i. cap. xiii.

All authors agree, that the whole body is affected, but
more particularly the ftomach and belly, and the head by
confent. The *cardialgia, fingultus,* and in fome the retention of the excretions, plainly fhew it.

Etiamfi

is a paffion of the body, not of the mind. That it is the effect of the bite, cannot in the leaft be doubted; but, moreover, that the mind alfo partakes of this effect, is as un-doubtedly true: and fuch is the alteration to be obferved therein, that either dejec-tion, melancholy, or furious madnefs, are the conftant attendants of it; which fhews, that the nerves and *fenforium commune* are ftrongly affected.

But the *hydrophobia* is not always a conco-mitant fymptom, although the difeafe excited by the bite of a mad dog fhould end fatally. The pain, fever, *delirium*, and convulfions, have appeared fucceffively, and deftroyed the patient on the third day, without the leaft fign of the *hydrophobia*, as Doctor MEAD acquaints us *. And profeffor BOERHAAVE attributes " the variety of appearance and effects of this " contagious *faliva*, both with regard to the " time it breaks out, and its various fymp- " toms, to the feafon of the year, the dif- " ferent degree of the difeafe in the furious " animal, the conftitution of the perfon " bitten, bilious habits being the moft ea- " fily affected, phlegmatic and dropfical the " leaft; and alfo to the feveral kinds of

---

Etiamfi rabie correptis, omnia excrementorum genera, ut plurimùm retineantur. In uno tamen vidi, maximam, & ingentem urinæ copiam, excretam, fine ullo ægrotantis fenfu. LISTER Exercit. p. 154.

* MEAD's Effays, p. 147.

" food,

" food, and to the medicines which are ad-
" miniftred *.

The *hydrophobia* is a fymptom common to
other difeafes †; it frequently attends the
phrenzy, and efpecially in hot countries. The
fentiments of HIPPOCRATES and ARETÆUS
have already been quoted.

‖ COELIUS AURELIANUS defines the phrenzy to be a diforder of the *meninges*, or membranes of the brain. Thefe membranes ferve
as coverings to the nerves, and of courfe cannot be affected, without communicating the
difeafe, in fome degree, to the brain, and to
fuch of the nerves as are contiguous to the feat
of the complaint; or by their connexion and
fympathy are liable to the fame impreffion :
whatever, therefore, caufes an irritation on
the *meninges*, an inflammation, a fever, fpafmodic contractions, or tenfion; whether it be
an ardent fever raifed by the obftruction of
perfpiration, or by a tranflation of matter,
called *metaftafis*, or a fudden ftoppage of the
lochia, or *menfes*, or by any fudden paffion of
the mind, fuch as anger, or fear; any of
thefe caufes may produce a phrenzy; and
from a communication of the fpafmodic con-

---

* Pendet vero hæc diverfitas, a calore tempeftatis anni,
a vario gradu morbi, in animali mordente, a temperie ho-
minis morfi, quum biliofi, eo facilius vergant, pituitofi, &
hydropici contra a diverfo victu, medicamentis adhibitis,
BOERHAAVII Aphorifm. 1137.

† VAN SWIETEN Comment. tom. iii. p. 537.

‖ COELIUS AURELIANUS, lib. i. cap. i. & feq.

vulfions,

vulfions, may, to the other fymptoms, add alfo the *hydrophobia.*

In thefe temperate climates, difeafes of fo violent a nature are not fo frequent as in hot countries; and whenever they do appear, their progrefs is not fo fpeedy; which may be the reafon why HIPPOCRATES had not an opportunity of feeing the intire *hydrophobia,* either in phrenitics, or perfons bitten by mad animals; the illnefs deftroying them on the firft appearance of the difficulty of fwallowing; whence they were called βραχυπόται, *parvibibuli.* The few inftances, therefore, which are met with in thefe climates, it cannot be improper to relate. The appearance of that terrible fymptom in feveral difeafes, and the inftances, however few, in which remedies have been applied with fuccefs, may take off from that univerfal dread, and fhew that it is not always incurable.

In *April* 1758, a farmer and grafier, about 40 years of age, of a fanguine conftitution, was feized with a violent pain a little above the *pubis*; an inflammation on the neck of the bladder, and total ftoppage of urine, enfued. He was bled, purged, and lenient diuretics were given him. The fymptoms abated upon a difcharge of purulent matter, which fhewed that the inflammation had terminated in an abfcefs. On the third of *May* the man, having fome evenings before taken cold by going after fome cattle in the wet, was again feized

D 3 with

with the fame fymptoms, but to a greater degree of violence; the fuppreffion of urine was
alfo total, and to a high fever and *delirium*
fucceeded a phrenzy, and fuch a furious madnefs, as to equal the moft difordered perfon.
In this fituation I found him when Mr. LITCH-
FIELD, an ingenious furgeon and apothecary
at *Ramfey*, in the county of *Huntingdon*, firft
fent for me. To all the figns of madnefs of
the moft mifchievous kind it muft be added,
that in his lucid intervals, which were chiefly
in the morning, he could not on the fifth and
fixth of *May* fwallow the leaft drop of liquid:
he grew outrageous at the prefenting it, fpit-
ting in the faces of his neareft relations, as well
as others, and telling them they meant to choak
him. By plentiful and repeated bleedings,
and emollient clyfters, bladders half filled
with warm water and milk, and applied to the
pubis, fomentations, *pediluvia*, fhaving his
head, and wafhing it with a lotion of *elder-
flower* water with *vinegar* and *camphor*, the
convulfive fpafms and the phrenzy were abated.
Oily and *terebinthinate* clyfters were injected,
and when a paffage could be had, lubricating,
cooling, laxative, and diuretic medicines were
adminiftred, which removed the complaint.
But, as he had been unavoidably brought low
by the repeated evacuations, it was a long time
before he recovered a fettled ftate of mind;
which, however, returned perfectly, by means
of the *cortex Peruvianus*, with proper refto-
ratives,

ratives, and change of air. At firſt the blood, I ſaw drawn from this perſon, was very black as it ran out; when cold, the grumous part was of a looſe texture, and the ſerous part an entire cake of purulent jelly containing it. This appearance in the blood, was certainly a proof of the *metaſtaſis*, or tranſlation of matter from the bladder, which had cauſed all the terrible effects before related.

Doctor MEAD quotes from SCHENCKIUS, that the " *hydrophobia* has been remarked in " malignant fevers;" and from the *Epheme-rides Germanicæ*, that " a melancholy has " ended fatally by this ſymptom." And this learned and experienced phyſician has ſeen " the *hydrophobia* laſt many hours in an hy-" ſteric diſorder, and in a caſe attended with " fits of a palpitation of the heart, wherein " the violence of the ſymptom ſeemed not to " differ from the true *hydrophobia*."

That this ſymptom is common to nervous diſeaſes, is alſo Doctor MEAD's opinion *. The ſuffocation called the *globus hyſtericus*, and ſo frequently met with in hyſterical caſes, has been produced, and increaſed to the *hy-drophobia*, upon a ſuppreſſion of the *menſes*, or of the *lochia*. I attended a young girl of ſixteen years of age, of a plethoric conſtitution, who from a ſuppreſſion of the *menſes*, on their

* MEAD, Eſſay on poiſons, p. 147.

firſt

firſt imperfect appearance, had all the hyſterical ſymptoms, to the higheſt degree : they
were followed by a *mania*, which laſted ſome
days. During this, ſhe had a difficulty of
ſwallowing*, and the *hydrophobia* two or
three days, which was removed by plentiful
bleedings, both in the foot and arm, and by
ſemicupia and glyſters ; but until the courſe of
the *menſes* became regular, ſhe was periodically
diſordered every month, ſo that ſhe could not
be deemed rightly in her ſenſes till that time.

I ſhall have occaſion hereafter to mention
another caſe, owing to the ſudden ſuppreſſion
and retention of the *lochia*, when I come to
ſhew the fatal conſequences ariſing from the
turbulent paſſions of the mind.

In the Medical Eſſays, Doctor INNES has
recorded, very circumſtantially, the caſe of a
young gentleman who had an inflammation
of the ſtomach, attended with the *hydrophobia* †. Although the young lady who was
under my care, and of whom I have given an
account in the Philoſophical Tranſactions ‖,
had not only a difficulty of ſwallowing, but
a total ſtoppage, ſo that the leaſt drop of any
liquid could not be admitted into the ſtomach,

---

* See Doctor ECCLES's Account of a great difficulty in
Swallowing and *Tetanus*, in the Medical Eſſays, vol. v.
part ii. p. 472.

† Medical Eſſays, vol. i. art. xxix. p. 283.

‖ Philoſophical Tranſactions, Nº 495.

nor,

nor, at times, far into the *œfophagus*; yet fhe had no dread at the fight of water, or of any fluid. The evacuations which fhe had undergone, before I attended her, might have prevented that degree of acrimony which was the caufe of the *hydrophobia* in Doctor INNES's cafe, where the cure was at length effected by repeated bleedings, and a fpontaneous vomiting.

* In that kind of catarrhal flux from the falival glands, and diftenfion of the lymphatic veffels, which, from the feat of the diforder, the *bronchi*, is called the *brancks*, or more ufually the mumps, and chiefly affects young perfons about the age of puberty; upon taking cold, or an improper treatment, the ferous matter is often tranflated from the throat to the tefticles, which grow hard, and the *fcrotum* is much enlarged, and becomes painful, through its weight: unlefs this fymptom be alfo carefully attended to, a tranflation of acrid matter is fometimes, by a fudden *metaftafis*, thrown upon the membranes of the brain, and this tranflation is followed by a fever, *delirium*, phrenzy, fpafms, and convulfions; which, if not timely remedied, will prove fatal. Such a fuffocation as the *globus hyftericus*, is generally obferved to be one of the fymptoms;

* HOFFMANNI Confultationes Medicinales, tom. ii. cafus cii. De teft um confenfu cum cerebro.

and

and from the fpafmodic contractions of the
mufcles of the throat, a difficulty of fwallowing renders fuch patients what HIPPO-
CRATES calls them, βραχυπόται, *parvibibuli,*
fmall drinkers; whenever this difeafe, as
COELIUS AURELIANUS obferves, is attended
with a ftricture, or tenfion, not in cafe of a
relaxation: both which different effects of
ftricture, tenfion, or relaxation, appear in
this illnefs. In fouthern climates the tranflation oftner occurs than in northern countries. The firft time I faw it to any confiderable degree, was in the fpring of
1760, when it appeared like an epidemical
difeafe affecting the private foldiers, and
chiefly the married men, belonging to both
the battalions of the *Effex* militia, quartered
in the county of *Huntingdon,* during the
months of *February, March,* and *April,*
particularly. The feafon, no doubt, prevented the violence of the fymptoms, which
would neceffarily have followed in a hotter
time of the year. I vifited feveral with
Mr. GORDON, who attended as furgeon to
the firft battalion: none died, although fome
were in a high fever; and one of my private patients was delirious. Agreeable to
this, is the doctrine of the venerable HIP-
POCRATES *, concerning the fympathy between feveral parts of the human body; and
TULPIUS, on another occafion, not very fo-

* HIPPOCRATES Περὶ τροφῆ; De Alimento.

reign

reign to the prefent inquiry, gives the following excellent caution *.

" Let it therefore be carefully inquired by
" phyficians, what kind of humor nature ex-
" pells, and let them be ftrictly on their guard
" that it doth not overflow, left it fhould fhift
" from a place of little moment, to a more
" noble and confiderable part."

The intimate and ftrict connection between
the body and the mind, although inexpreffi-
ble to our limited conceptions, is nevertheless
fo evident from its effects, as not in the leaft
to be doubted. Thus the difeafes of the body
influence the operations of the mind, and the
feveral paffions of the mind, either promote,
difturb, fufpend, or deftroy the natural functions, and the fecretions of the human body,
according to the different powers the feveral
paffions have allotted them. Joy dilates, ex-
hilarates and circulates the blood with the moft
agreeable fenfation. Grief relaxes, debilitates
and fufpends the neceffary ftreams of life. The
tender paffions of love and friendfhip warm
the blood, and give it frefh vigor. The turbulent paffions, on the contrary of wrath and
fear contract the veffels, and hurry the circulation of the blood in fo violent a manner, as
to throw the whole frame into confufion.

* Inquirendum itaque curiofe, medicis, in naturam hu-
moris a natura expulfi, & cavendum obnixe, ne facili re-
gurgitet, a loco ignobili, in partem principem. Tulpii
Obferv. medicinal. lib. i. cap. ix.

When-

Whenever thefe two wrath and fear are raifed
together, there is a terrible fcene produced, if
an inftantaneous death doth not end the tragedy by a fudden apoplexy; a palfy, a phrenzy, or
epilepfy, follow in fanguine conftitutions; convulfions, tremors, *fchirrus*, cancers and many
weakneffes attend thofe of a lax and cacochy-
mic habit of body.   But the limits of this effay will not allow me to expatiate farther on
thefe particulars, I fhall therefore confine myfelf to the remarking only by a very ftrong inftance the fatal effects of the violent paffions
of † wrath and fear operating alternately and
jointly in the fame perfon.—An inftance in
which not only a phrenzy, but what is much
to our prefent purpofe, a total alteration of the
fluids, and an *hydrophobia* were produced.

A young woman about 27 years of age, of
a fair complexion, delicate conftitution, good
habit of body, of a lively and fweet temper,
but rather of a timorous difpofition; in child-
bed of her fourth child, was on the eighth day
from her delivery, in a fair way of recovery,
and receiving the ufual congratulations of her fe-
male acquaintance. Among other vifitors came
a relation with whom there had been fome fa-

---

† Doctor GEORGE BAKER in his differtation *De affec-*
tibus animi mentions the feveral opinions of poets, and of
philofophers ‡, anger was looked upon as a temporary
madnefs, and the fpafmodic contractions through fear are
elegantly defcribed ‖.

‡ GALEN, HORATIUS, lib. i. Epift. ii. Ira furor brevis eft.
‖ LUCRETIUS, &c.

mily

mily difputes. This perfon very unfeafonably revived the quarrel, and after the moft aggravating provocation infulted the lying-in woman with the moft bitter invectives and moft opprobrious language. The by-ftanders fearing that even words would not fatisfy her revenge, with great difficulty removed her out of the room; but irreparable mifchief was already done. Anger and fear had been raifed fo ftrongly in the mind of the patient, that unable to retort any longer to the revilings of her adverfary fhe fell into a violent hyfteric fit, little inferior to the higheft degree of an epilepfy *.

The *lochia* inftantly ftopped, the milk difappeared, a fuffocation, fever, and phrenzy enfued. Early next morning I was fent for, and immediately had her blooded plentifully in the foot, *pediluvia* and clyfters were ufed, and deobftruent boluffes given; although fhe attempted feveral times, not a drop of liquid could be fwallowed on account of the frequent fpafmodic contractions. Blifters were applied to the thighs and legs; the head was fhaved and wafhed with a lotion of *camphorated vinegar* and *elder flower* water, but all my endeavors proved ineffectual. The tenfion was fo

---

* Nonnulla etiam excrementa quæ in utilitatem vitæ noftræ inftituit providens natura fufcepto metu, fifti protinus, & ceffare, res eft medentibus nimium familiaris. Notum eft, nimis quam gravis fit ille puerperæ, lactanti que, abortus fcilicet inde nafci, cum læthali hæmorrhagia, fifti lochia, coire lac, &c. BAKER de affectibus animi, p. 17.

great,

great, that neither opiates, *camphor*, nitre, nor repeated applications of bladders filled half full with warm water and milk, and applied to the *hypogaftric* region could relax. The nervous contractions increafed fo faft, that general convulfions fucceeded with fuch perturbations of mind upon their remiffion, that the leaft fight of a pellucid object, the light, the leaft noife or ruftling of cloths alarmed her with the fear of her relations return. Thus fhe continued three days. A few hours before her death fhe recovered her fenfes, but could neither fwallow nor bear the fight of liquids; fhe then knew me, and told me that fhe doubted not I had done my utmoft to fave her, but that it was to no purpofe; and laying her hand upon her heart, added, that fhe was wounded too deeply there.

A fymptom not to be forgotten, and which fhewed the violence of the fever, was, that no urine was difcharged but by force, at the time of her convulfions when they were the ftronger, and then it was as a jelly of the moft tenacious kind. The celebrated profeffor HOFFMANN *, has recorded the violent effects of anger and fear in feveral of his obfervations, and imputes the appearance of the various fymptoms to the irregular circulation, and

* HOFFMANNI Confultationes medicinales. De terroris indole, tom. i. p. 20. cafus vii. De terrore in puerperiis, tom. i. p. 196. cafus xxxvii. De effectu terroris, & iræ, tom. ii. p. 225. cafus xlvii, &c.

want

want of a due fecretion of the fluids, which the paffions of the mind fuddenly bring on; and his prefcriptions all tend towards the removing the tenfion and obftruction.

Thus from the feveral inftances prod ced from authors and others juft related, the *hydrophobia* appears to be a fymptom common to feveral difeafes, and particularly in cafes attended with fpafmodic contractions of the nerves of the throat, and increafed by the violent paffions of the mind, chiefly anger and fear. The fight of liquids or of any pellucid object, equally act on the unhappy perfon, whatever be the caufe that produces the pain; for the admiffion of liquids in the leaft quantity conveys down the *œfophagus* into the ftomach, the putrid, acrid *faliva*, which irritates the upper orifice * and nervous coat of the ftomach, and the *œfophagus* already inflamed, the *mucus* being dried up by the conftant fwallowing of the acrid particles; the fight alfo of a glafs, of a white wall, or a glaring light ftriking ftrongly upon the *fenforium commune*, awakens the remembrance of the accident which has happened, and revives all the terrors which the bite of a mad animal had occafioned †. The

---

* At falivam deglutire, ei horrendum fecit, perinde ac fi mortem ipfo momento inferret. Vide hiftoriam JACOBI CORTON in exercit. iiiᵃ. LISTERI p. 117.

† There be fights that are horrible, becaufe they excite the memory of things that are odious and fearful. BACON's fylva fylvarum experiments touching, pleafing or difpleafing the fenfes, cent. vii. § 700.

hydro-

hydrophobia *, therefore, is a conftant atten-
dant upon fuch acute difeafes, as are dangerous
through ftricture and tenfion ; and more particularly in the bite of a mad dog.   Whenever
this fevere fymptom appears, it is the more fatal ; the greater the tenfion and inflammation,
the longer the fymptom has lafted ; and from
the different rigidity of the fibres, it is by far
more difficult to remove in men than women.
The figns of its approach, and the fymptoms
that ufually attend it, have been fufficiently
defcribed in the former fection.

  * Hydrophobia eft morbus acutus.   LISTER exercitatio
iii². p. 106.

SECTION III.

Of the different Methods of Cure.

THE different methods of cure, for the effects arifing from the bite of a mad dog, are either rational or empirical.

By the rational is to be underftood, the internal adminiftration or external application of fuch remedies; which by experience, are found to remove or prevent the complaint in certain conftitutions and circumftances of the diftemper, and whofe efficacy, may in a great meafure be accounted for, by arguments founded upon obfervation, and according to the known power of medicines without the leaft prefumption of their being infallible.

By the empirical cure, I underftand the indifcriminate ufe of any *noftrum* or known medicine, in all degrees of the fame illnefs, adminiftered or applied to all conftitutions and fexes, and in all ages, with a pofitive affurance of an infallibility, and whofe operations are not only of a violent, and dangerous, or wholly infignificant nature, but will neither bear the teft of examination by reafoning, nor a fcrutiny into their fuccefs, the cafes being frequently mifreprefented, or the fatal confequences fuppreffed.

E   It

It muſt be owned, that mere accident has produced both in the early days of practice; and medicine hath gained great advantages from the obſervation of, and a due attention to, the *juvántia* and *lædentia*. Thus a rational method of cure, took its riſe from accident, preſumption and empiriciſm.

Was the world, with all its improvements in this enlightened age, ſufficiently guarded againſt impoſitions, there would be no longer a neceſſity of dwelling upon the conſideration of ſuch abſurdities, as are ſo many reproaches to the human underſtanding; but while through tradition, plauſible authority, or preſumptuous practitioners, mankind is ſtill deluded, it behoves every one, who has the welfare of his fellow-creatures at heart, to point out to them the dangers which they run, by confiding in an empirical rather than a rational method of cure.

The plea of empirics is, that ſeldom doth any diſtemper appear in any perſon, as deſcribed by any ſyſtematical writer, and therefore facts are only to be relied on. Certainly, many circumſtances may occur, to vary the appearance of an illneſs in different conſtitutions and ſituations; but whoever is furniſhed with a ſummary of the ſeveral ſymptoms of a diſeaſe, will be the readier to relieve the diſtreſſed, than by following indiſcriminately the ſame method in every caſe, becauſe he ſaw it ſucceed in one.

Syſtems

Syftems unfupported by facts, are fruitlefs *hypothefes*; but when reafon and experience agree, although they will never be infallible, yet they will jointly afford the greateft proba=bility of fuccefs.

Both the rational and empirical methods, may be divided into the preventive or the actual cure. I fhall begin with the empirical method.

And firft, the moft dangerous and abfurd notion ftill prevailing in fome diftant ages, is, that if a perfon bitten by a mad dog, can immediately get the liver of the dog, and eat it raw or broiled, it is a means to prevent the progrefs of the difeafe. Every author, now a days, judicioufly pronounces, that fuch a di=ftempered liver is neither good for food or phy=fic †, the bile contained in it being of the moft vitiated kind; and although it has not yet been difcovered, whether fuch bilious falts admitted into the ftomach have only like other putrid humors produced a *naufea* and *diarbœa*; or, if paffing into the blood, they have excited the fame madnefs, as the bite of a mad dog; one may venture to declare an utter abhorrence of fuch food, and that it can be of no other account, than as it may procure fome quiet to the patient's mind, by laying afleep for the prefent his apprehenfions of the ufual confe=quences.

† MEAD's Effay on poifons, p. 158.

Thefe

Thefe notions which Doctor LISTER calls the fuperftitious fancies of ancient times, feem to prevail ftill in *Ireland*, among the lower fort of people, and to obviate the repetition of fuch a fhocking fcene, as was related in a letter from *Gallaway*, inferted in the public news-papers, and dated the 11th of *February* 1760, I have been the more ferious to explode fuch an abfurd practice. I will relate the material circumftances of the horrid tragedy in the moft tender manner poffible.

" A gentleman in the neighbourhood of
" *Slave Muree*, in the county of *Gallaway*,
" writes word. That a young man, who had
" been bitten by a mad dog, almoft three years
" before, was married to a young woman of
" *Slave Muree*, and the very night of their nup-
" tials, the relations alarmed at the cries of
" the woman, burft into the room and found
" him with her liver in his teeth. A knife
" in his hand, and his wild afpect not to be
" defcribed, would not permit any one to ap-
" proach him; and to prevent further mur-
" der, his own brother was tempted to fhoot
" him; but he was fecured by a noofe thrown
" over his neck, and tied down."

This cafe plainly fhews the neceffity of putting a ftop to fuch a dangerous notion; for no doubt, his imagination being heated, and the latent *virus* breaking forth, brought to his mind the reprefentation of the dog, whom in the rage of phrenzy, he thought he was deftroying;
and

and that, with the prepoffeffion of curing himfelf, by eating of his liver.

. The curd of a fucking puppy's milk, or the
hair of the mad dog intended as a cure for the
wound he gave, are applications to be laughed at.

The next ridiculous and idle tale, is the
boafted effects from the prefenting a *Hyæna*'s
fkin to the perfon bitten, or tying a piece of
the fame creature's fkin in a linen rag on the
wounded limb. The notion, it is faid, takes
it's rife from an averfion dogs have naturally
for *Hyænas*; from whence it is ftrongly con-
jectured, that this canine diftemper fhould be
removed on the fight or touch of the *Hyæna*'s
fkin, and the venom at once frighted away by
this fort of amulet.

The root of the *cynorrhodon*, the dog-rofe,
is now thought of no efficacy, although PLINY
extolled it much; nor is much ftrefs laid on
the other properties of the *fpongia cynorrhodi*, the
fponge of the *dog rofe*; but this fhall be mentioned in fpeaking of the rational procefs of cure.

Among the empirical jumbles not to be
trufted to, are the feveral *theriaca* *, confec-
tions, and fpecific antidotes hitherto recommended, to expell this poifonous venom, and
which would much more fpeedily and effectually affift the mifchievous effects of it.

Nor are family *noftrums* of any kind to lull
any perfon into a fatal fecurity, for they are

* See Doctor HEBERDEN's Effay on the *Mithridatium*
and *Theriaca.*

E 3   gene-

generally nothing more than mutilated copies of prefcriptions tranfcribed full of errors, and frequently directed for an oppofite intention, notwithftanding the fanction of being care-fully handed down, from year to year, in the fame families.

I now proceed to the rational cure. This confifts in fuch external applications, or in-ternal remedies, as are adminiftred, either to prevent the progrefs of the inoculated *faliva*, that it may not fpread it's infection, or to re-move the bad effects of the poifonous *virus*, when it has already infinuated itfelf fo far, as to produce the greateft mifchiefs, and endan-ger the patient's life.

In the examination of the feveral methods directed, I fhall endeavor to account for the intention of each practice.

Firft, In order to extract the *faliva* which by the bite may have been depofited in the wound. The ancients advifed the application of ‖ cupping-glaffes †, to draw out the *faliva*; and made a plentiful difcharge of blood by applying the *fcarificator* : but this operation will not infure the removal of the *faliva*.

Nor will the fucking of the wound *, to extract the *faliva* of a mad animal, be either fafe, or to be depended upon : for although the venomous *faliva* of vipers has been fucked,

‖ Celsus, lib. v. cap. 27.
† Palmarius, p. 336.
* Ibid. p. 338.

and

and received into the ſtomach without any bad effect; yet it remains doubtful, whether that *ſaliva* lodged in a carious tooth, or admitted into any the ſmalleſt wound, in the mouth, would not be attended with fatal ſymptoms; much more imprudent would it be, to apply the mouth to the bite of a mad dog, whoſe *ſaliva*, once admitted among the glands, or into the leaſt wound, might produce the dreadful diſeaſe: and in this operation there is not a certainty of extracting the poiſon to authoriſe ſuch a dangerous practice.

REDI, in his Natural experiments on the poiſonous effects of the *ſaliva* of a viper, p. 263. ſays, that the admiſſion of the poiſon depends on the ſort of wound made: if too ſmall, the *virus* will hardly penetrate; if too large, the effuſion of blood will be ſo conſiderable, as to bring away the poiſonous *ſaliva* along with it. Hence appears the uſe of immediate ſcarifications, without cupping, where the part will allow of them.

Secondly, To inlarge the wound, either by dilatation, or by taking the piece out which the dog had bitten, ſeemed a ſurer way of diſlodging the poiſonous *ſaliva*; but, as Doctor MEAD obſerves, the ſeverity of ſuch a practice is needleſs; ſince it cannot always be done in time, nor can it be known whether the *ſaliva* has made any impreſſion, or not.

The ſame may be ſaid of cauteries, whether actual, or potential; ſuch as a red-hot

iron

iron, cauftics*, corrofive or irritating ointments, blifters, or drawing plaifters ‖ ; whofe
application is more painful and terrifying to
the patient than promifing, in it's confequences
of fuccefs †. Iffues are recommended, by
Ætius, to be kept a long while open.

Some have advifed the rubbing a pickle of
falt and *vinegar* on the wound ; Doctor Parsons has lately recommended it : and the
Rev. Dr. Jared Elliott has feen the fuccefs of it in *New England* and *Connecticut.*
A furgeon of Doctor Parsons's acquaintance,
alfo, has fuccefsfully made ufe of the *fpirit* of
falt with the fame intention, to refift acrimony and putrefaction. Others have wafhed
the wound with a *lixivium* of *oak afhes* and
urine.

Emollient cataplafms of *bread* and *milk,*
either by themfelves, or together with opiates,
as the *theriaca,* or pure *opium,* have been laid
on the wound to affuage the pain, decreafe
the irritation, and relax the fibres. Others
have made pultices of *forrel, rue,* roafted
onions, bruifed *garlic, leeks, yeaft, muftard feed*
and *falt,* and *oil* of *fcorpions,* to irritate the
wound, and caufe a difcharge of the poifonous *faliva.* Some have anointed the part
with *oil* and pure *wine* mixed together, or
have wafhed it with fat broth. And the *anus*

---

* Lister, Exercitatio iii[a], p. 136.
‖ Palmarius, p. 337.
† Freind Opera, p. 146.

of an old cock is directed to be put to the wound, to draw out the *virus* *.

† Bleeding, even till the perfon is faint, has been practifed with great fuccefs, efpecially in fanguine and plethoric conftitutions, to remove the fulnefs and irritation, and to prevent the ftricture and tenfion, both as a preventive cure, and in the confirmed ftate of the illnefs; and yet fome difapprove of bleeding, at firft, left the *virus* fhould be drawn in, from the external parts, to circulate with the blood all over the body.

So generally has almoft every nation adopted the notion, that the immerfion, or plunging the perfon bitten into the fea, is an infallible cure, that whoever has been found to controvert it, has feldom been hearkened to: but, among other inftances which might be produced of the inefficacy of this cuftom, and that the only advantage accruing from it, is to quiet the perfon's mind who has been bitten; Doctor DESAULT relates ‖, that his uncle DAUBAIGNAN, and DUFOURC his fellow ftudent, both died mad, although they were both dipped in the fea, and went to the fea-

---

* PALMARIUS, p. 337.
Philofophical Tranfactions, N° 191. p. 140.
† SPEED Commentarius de Aqua marina, p. 25.
Doctors HARTLEY and SANDYS account of a perfon cured of the *rabies canina* by lofing 120 ounces of blood, Philofophical Tranfactions, N° 448.
‖ DESAULT Differtation fur la rage, p. 287, 288.

fhore

fhore the very next day after they had received
the bite: and adds, that he could eafily fwell
the bulk of his Differtation, were he to mention the great number of unfortunate perfons
to whom bathing, or, as he defcribes it, forcibly plunging *, into the fea, was of no fort
of ufe.

Immerfions are recommended and firft
mentioned by CELSUS †, who fays, " It is
" the only remedy;" and advifes to " throw
" the perfon unawares into water, and, if he
" cannot fwim, to be kept under water, that
" he may fwallow it, and then, at times, be
" lifted out of it; if he can fwim, to hold
" him under by force, that he may drink,
" whether he will, or not: by thefe means
" the thirft and dread of water will be re-
" moved at the fame time."

As CELSUS makes ufe of the word *pifcinam*, a fifh-pond, or pool of water; it is
plain, he means frefh, not falt water. VAN
HELMONT ‖, in the beginning of the laft
century, obferving the good effects of plunging in the fea in *Flanders*, ftrongly recom-

---

* Ibid. p. 288.

† Unicum remedium eft, nec opinantem, in pifcinam
non ante ei provifam projicere, & fi natandi fcientiam non
habet modò merfum bibere pati, modo attollere; fi habet,
interdum deprimere, ut invitus quoque aqua fatietur. Sic
enim fimul, & fitis, & aquæ metus tollitur. CELSUS,
lib. v. cap. 27.

‖ VAN HELMONT, Ortus Medicinæ.

mends

mends the practice; and Monfieur MORIN relates ‡, that a young girl, of 20 years of age, had all the fymptoms of madnefs, which appeared fixteen days after her being bitten in the hand, by a little boy who was mad, and was brought to bear the fight of water, without emotion, by being plunged into a bath made of river water, rather cold than hot, in which a bufhel of falt had been diffolved. Nothing extraordinary followed; a fever came on, which was treated in the common method: fhe took emetics, continued the ufe of bathing, and was cured.

One would imagine that CELSUS had two intentions in his method of immerfion: firft, by throwing the patient into water unprepared, and unexpectedly to caufe fuch a furprize as would give a ftrong fhock to the human frame; fecondly, by half drowning him, to make him fwallow a quantity of water before the *hydrophobia* comes on.

From the naufeous tafte of fea water, the awful appearance of the fea, and the approach of it's roaring billows, ftrong effects may arife, in a perfon who never faw the fea before; and more efpecially, if in the moft terrifying and forcible manner they are plunged, and half drowned. The fea water is never fo cold as frefh water is, and therefore cannot act on the fibres with the fame conftriction

‡ Hiftoire de l'Academie Royale des Sciences, année 1699.

which

which attends the immerſion in cold ſpring or river water. By its acrid taſte it will occaſion vomiting and purging, and the ſhock which the nerves have ſuſtained by the plunging, together with the ſtrong impreſſion left on the mind, will cauſe a conſiderable revolution in the humors of the human body, and help to diſlodge the remaining active ſalts, after the firſt paſſages have been cleared of the vitiated *ſaliva* and bile which load and irritate the ſtomach *.

But, notwithſtanding theſe advantages attending the dipping in the ſea, accidents may happen which will deter the moſt ſanguine from following CELSUS's advice of bathing either in the ſea, or otherwiſe, if the perſon is to be plunged unexpectedly, or forcibly.

The following inſtance, communicated to me by a perſon of credit, will ſhew how cautiouſly ſuch attempts are to be made; ſince, like the old and abſurd cuſtom of affrighting perſons by throwing them unawares into water, or by ſome other ſurprize, in the caſe of intermitting fevers, the patient has been freed, indeed, from one diſorder; but, at the ſame time, ſubjected to another, no leſs terrible and calamitous.

This gentleman was, during his ſtudies at *Oxford*, intimately acquainted with another

---

* At cum *ſaliva* venenata præcipuè noxia ſit, illa imprimis evacuanda temperandaque ne ſtomachum amplius offendat. LISTER, Exercitatio iii[a] p. 136.

ſtudent,

ftudent, of the fame college, who was of an amiable, and chearful, but of a modeft and rather timid difpofition of mind. He was one day bitten by his favorite cat, which was fuppofed to have been bitten by a mad dog, and inftantly, without allowing time for examining the creature, was declared mad, and killed. The young gentleman was then hurried away to the fea, and, as ufual, forcibly plunged into it feveral times, out of which he was taken half drowned, and with this fuccefs, that no fymptom of madnefs, or of an *hydrophobia*, appeared; but he became mopifh, and ftupid, and continued fo till his death, which happened three years after the immerfion.

Doctor LISTER has recorded*, from the authority of ARDOYN and of Doctor THOROUGHTON of *Nottingham*, that fome perfons have been fuffocated by plunging them into water againft their will: and I am favored with the following cafe by a phyfician of great rank and eminence, who not only remembers the fact, but faw Doctor ASHENHURST's written account of it.

A man, who was bitten by a mad dog, became mad, and had the *hydrophobia* on the approach of the full moon, and was ordered by the late Doctor ASHENHURST, of *Cambridge*, to be plunged into the cold bath near

* LISTER loc. cit.

SIR

Sir John Hinde Cotton's feat at *Maddingley* in that neighbourhood. The firft immerfion freed the patient of both the *hydrophobia* and madnefs. A month after, on the return of thefe fymptoms, he was again plunged, and once more relieved: but, upon relapfing a third time, at the next full moon, and his being again put into the cold bath, he was feized with a total diftenfion of the nerves, and immediately died convulfed in the water.

Doctor Speed *, who has wrote a very judicious and elegant commentary on fea water, tells us, that it has been a cuftom long fince, to bathe in the fea for the bite of a mad dog: and that, provided the perfons bitten bathe before the madnefs comes on, it often anfwers; but after it's appearance, bathing in the fea is never to be relied on. The Doctor adds, that he has by him the cafe of a girl, who, in the year 1707, having the *hydrophobia* ftrongly upon her from the bite of a mad cat, was perfectly cured by frequent fcarifications of the wound, repeated bleedings, blifters, purgatives, and fudorifics: but as neither in this cafe, nor in any other, in the courfe of that great experience which Doctor Speed, and his father, muft have had of the utility of fea bathing, any mention is made of it's efficacy; it feems probable, that the boafted cures performed in this illnefs by fea water, have been wrought on fuch perfons who have repaired

* Speed Commentarius de Aqua marina, p. 24.

to

to the fea fhore, fuppofing themfelves in great danger, when the dog, who bit them, may have never been mad. Undoubtedly cures fo remarkable, and of fo much confequence to fociety, would not have efcaped Doctor SPEED's notice.

To Doctor DESAULT's teftimony of the inefficacy of fea bathing, for the preventing the *hydrophobia*, at or near *Bourdeaux*, may be added, the obfervation of Monfieur CLAUDE DU CHOISEL *, a *Jefuit*, and apothecary to the miffion of *French Jefuits* at *Pondicherry*. His words are;

" Bathing in the fea has hitherto been " looked upon as an infallible prefervative " againft the bite of a mad dog. The ex- " perience which I have had of it in all thofe " patients who were not treated according to " my new method, has proved to me the fal- " fity of that opinion. They bathed them- " felves every day in the fea, but to no pur- " pofe, not one of them furvived the bite " longer than thirty or three and thirty days. " I do not, however, difapprove of thofe " bathings, where they ferve to quiet the " minds of the patients. Befides, the *In-* " *dians* ufually bathe themfelves every day. " We are fituated here on the fea fhore, and " it is a matter of indifference whether a few " waves of fea water pafs over their bodies, or

* DU CHOISEL's Method of treating perfons bit by mad animals, p. 18.

" they

" they wafh themfelves in a pond. In this
" hot country there is no danger of obftructed
" perfpiration, or pleurifies. If I were at a
" greater diftance from the fea coaft, and in
" a cold country, I would have nothing to do
" with fuch fort of remedies, which I look
" upon as entirely ufelefs, in the cure of this
" difeafe."

Bathing in the fea has not, then, fuch advantages, as may not be procured by other
means. For if the chief be the emptying the
ftomach of the acrid bile, by the fwallowing
of the fea water, this operation can be much
more eafily performed: and as to the immerfion, the water is not cold enough; nor will
any one recommend the forcible plunging, for
the reafons above mentioned; and perfons will
be to the full as much fatisfied in their minds,
when they are convinced that an eafier method of cure is practifed than that of hurrying
them into the fea, where there is not the fame
probability of fuccefs.

Celsus * not only recommends bathing in
a pond as preventive cure, but even in the
violence of the *hydrophobia*: adding, however; " that care is to be taken left a tender
" conftitution, being affected by cold water,
" fhould be feized with a diftenfion of the

---

* Sed aliud periculum excipit, ne infirmum corpus in
aqua frigida vexatum, nervorum diftentio abfumat. Id ne
incidat a pifcina protinùs in oleam calidam demittendus eft.
Celsus, lib. v. cap. 27.

" nerves.

" nerves. To prevent which, fays he, let
" the perfon be inftantly conveyed from the
" pond into a bath of warm oil."

Profeffor BOERHAAVE, from CELSUS, directs cold bathing in the fame manner as
practifed by the ancients, or to throw cold
water on the perfon till the dread of water
ceafes. This method is thought to be rather
expofing the patient to a greater tenfion and
ftricture of the parts. Doctor MEAD recommends cold fpring or river water only as a preventive, and after bleeding to promote perfpiration, and a flux of urine. Profeffor HOFF-
MAN prefers the ufe of temperate baths, in all
ftrictures of the nervous parts, and moderate
draughts of wine, to promote the circulation
of the blood. The difference in opinion, between Doctor MEAD and profeffor HOFF-
MAN, with regard to cold or temperate bathing, may be reconciled by obferving, that they
are each directed in a different ftage of the
illnefs, and therefore are advifed to be ufed accordingly. The conftitution of the patient,
time of the year, but efpecially the fort of infection, whether putrid, or not, ought certainly to be attended to; and unlefs bathing
be cautioufly ordered, it will oftner prove
prejudicial, than falutary.

Internal medicines, of various kinds, were
prefcribed according to the practitioner's intention, either to prevent the ill effects of the

F   poi-

poifonous *faliva*, or with a view to expel it out of the body.

Thus, firft, to cool and quench the thirft, the herbs *purflane*, *wood forrel*, and *forrel*, were recommended ; alfo, *burnet*, *burnet faxifrage*, *rue*, and *chervil*, as diuretics ; *marigolds*, *borage*, and *mint*, to warm and ftimulate ; and *lettuce*, to procure fleep*. The plant and ftalk of *black currants* † is ftill looked upon in *Sweden* as no contemptible remedy in the *hydrophobia*. It is well known, that in fuch countries which are liable to putrid and bilious fevers, the infufion of *black currants* leaves is in great efteem ; and a jelly of thofe currants, made with fugar, is highly commended in contagious difeafes, and fome fore throats. That all vegetable acids correct the too violent acrimony of the bilious falts, is the opinion of BOERHAAVE, HOFFMAN, MEAD, HUXHAM, and almoft all modern phyficians ; but this is only a palliative cure. I therefore proceed,

Secondly, To confider the intentions for which more powerful remedies are adminiftred.

---

* PALMARIUS, p. 343.

† See Mr. JOHN GEORGE BEYERSTEIN's obftacles to the improvement of phyfic, in Mifcellaneous tracts tranflated from the Amænitates Academiæ Upfalenfis, by Mr. STILLINGFLEET, p. 173.

I. * Some

I. * Some were defigned to fheathe the humor, and carry it down ; as the *oil* of *rofes*, drank to five ounces † : as purgatives, the expreffed *oil* of *walnuts*, the nuts themfelves, and *hiera picra*. But the moft efficacious medicine, both as a purgative, and an emetic, and which has not only been greatly extolled by the ancients, but is ftill made ufe of, with fuccefs, to this day, and particularly for dogs, and other quadrupeds, is the *white hellebore* ‖ : one dram of this root, powdered, and drank in a draught of milk, or forced down, made up into a *bolus* with a little butter, has operated fo ftrongly, both as an emetic, and purge, as to carry off all the fymptoms which had appeared. The fooner it is given after the. bite is received, the lefs irritation is to be feared from it's operation ; but, left the patient

---

* *Oils* have been both recommended and forbidden even fo long as in GALEN's time. BAGLIVI condemns the too general ufe of *oil* in *Italy*; and BIANCHI fays, that he has known bilious fevers increafe after the *oil* of *fweet almonds* had been given. BARON VAN SWIETEN, in his Commentaries on BOERHAAVE's Aphorifms, declares, That the mildeft and fofteft *oil*, when fpoiled, is of the moft putrid nature. The fweeter *oil* of *almonds*, that is exprefled, grows fo rank and corrupted in a few days, as to become very fharp, and fcalds the throat while it is fwallowing down. Aphorifm 89. p. 130.

† LISTER loc. cit. & in hiftoria JACOBI CORTON.

‖ Illud quidem verum eft, hoc medicamentum pituitam vehementer movere, evacuareque, quæ cum falivæ venenatæ. proxima materia fit, fic fortè adjuvare poffit. LISTER.

DIOSCORIDES, lib. iv. cap. cl. & in Therlaca, cap. ii.

fhould

ſhould be too much weakened, the perſons who adviſe this root, caution their patients againſt bleeding.

I was informed by the late Mr. HENRY BLAINE, of *Hartford* near *Huntingdon*, who had experienced the effects of the *white helle-bore*, in many dogs, that he had ſuccesſfully adminiſtred it in all ſtages of the diſeaſe, nay, when the fury and *hydrophobia* was ſo ſtrong on the dog, that no one dare approach him : and the method he uſed was, to faſten the dog's head down between the prongs of a pitch fork, and then thruſt down the ball made of the powdered *hellebore* and butter. *Hellebore* is alſo given, by way of ſternutatory, or ehrine, in clyſters, and applied in the form of a ſuppoſitory.

PALMARIUS reports *, that dogs having taken *hellebore* with *polenta*, were vomited, and immediately relieved from their madneſs. This method, taken from DIOSCORIDES †, ariſes from a practice very common among the ancients, both *Greeks* and *Romans*, to drink large quantities of the *polenta*, to ſtrengthen their ſtomachs, and cure them of a *diarrhœa*. The *polenta* is a decoction of oat bread toaſted, in ſpring water, till it be of a brown color like coffee. PLINY ſays, that in his time it dif-

---

* Addunt nonnulli, canes rabioſos elleboro cum po-lenta accepto vomuiſſe, & ſtatim a rabie liberatos ad ſe re-diiſſe. PALMARIUS, p. 339.

† DIOSCORIDES loco citato.

fered

fered from barley meal in that it was much toafted, or parched, and fometimes the Romans mixed a little *linfeed* with it, fome *falt*, and *coriander* feed. It is mentioned by Hippo-crates *, Aretæus, and Paulus Ægi-neta; and efpecially recommended for the cure of the *cholera* †. Doctor Charles Ay-ton Douglas has revived the ufe of this de-coction in *Scotland*, and given an account of it's efficacy, both on himfelf, and others. Doctor Douglas orders it to be made out of bread baked without any leaven or yeaft, care-fully toafted as brown as coffee, but not burnt: as occafion requires, he fometimes adds wine to the decoction. Somewhat fimi-lar to this practice is the ufe of *barley water*, *toaft and water*, and *water gruel*, drank chiefly in ardent and bilious fevers; and from the preference which Doctor Tissot ‖ obferved his patients gave to *oatmeal*, agreeable to pro-feffor Boerhaave's opinion, it may be fairly concluded, that in the difeafe produced by the bite of a mad dog, the *polenta* will prove as efficacious as in the *cholera*.

Some have given an infufion of the leaves of *rue*, of the inner bark of *elder*, of the in-ner green bark of *box*, to vomit and purge

---

* Hippocrates De affectionibus.
Aretæus, lib. ii. cap. v. p. 102, 104.
Paulus Ægineta, lib. i. cap. lxxviii.
† Medical Effays, vol. v. part ii. N° lxv.
‖ Tissot Differtatio de febribus bilioris, p. 75.

dogs;

dogs; or thofe ingredients dried, and powdered, and made into cakes with flower and
milk.

Profeffor BOERHAAVE advifes clyfters of
falt water, with *nitre*, and a little *vinegar*, both
to purge, and cool.

II. The ancients, in order to expel poifons
through the pores of the fkin, had their *alexi-
pharmaca* and *theriaca*; the firft to remove the
poifons of the mineral or vegetable kind, and
the latter the poifonous *virus* of animals. For
thofe purpofes, they ordered all the warm
fpicy medicines they could colleƈt: not only
thofe renowned jumbles known by the name
of *mithridatium* and *theriaca*, but alfo the
pancake compofed of oyfter-fhells, *&c.* which
Doƈtor DESAULT records; the famous *Sici-
lian* antidote made by APULEIUS CELSUS,
and yearly fent over to *Sicily*, as SCRIBONIUS
LARGUS relates, were direƈted; but additions of the afhes of *frefh water crabs* *, calcined oyfter-fhells, and of the filings or powder
of *tin*, have been made, by way of precipi-
tating or difperfing the venomous particles.
The firft was recommended by GALEN, ORI-
BASIUS, ÆTIUS RUFUS, and POSIDONIUS;
and the *crabs* were direƈted to be calcined with
the tendereft twigs of the *white vine*; thefe
afhes were to be well fifted, and mixed with
the powder of *gentian* root, to which was

* DIOSCORIDES loco citato.

fometimes

fometimes added *frankincenfe*, as Dioscorides advifes *: but giving *tin* is of a later date, and was much extolled by Sir Theodore Mayern, and Doctor Grew, and is commonly known by the name of *the pewter medicine.* There is very little difference between this remedy, as defcribed in the Philofophical Tranfactions: Doctor Bates's *decoctum ad morfum canis rabidi*, and the *decoctum antilyffum* of Doctor Fuller; being compofed of filings of *tin*, of *garlic*, and *rue*, boiled in wine, or ftrong *ale*, to which is added *London* or *Venice treacle* and *mithridate*.

From the chief ingredients of thefe compofitions one may eafily conclude, that their efficacy was expected from their pungency and warmth. As prefervatives againft contagion, *garlic* and *rue* were anciently taken; all kinds of *treacles* and *mithridates* have been thought to expel venom; and *tin* has been looked upon as a certain *vermifuge*; but yet no reliance is to be made upon thefe preparations, to remove the effects arifing from the bite of a mad dog.

III. The next intention feems to have been to difcharge the poifonous *virus* through the urinary paffages by means of diuretics. With this view was the *fpongia cynorrhodi*, or fponge of the *dog-rofe*, directed; which, from its efficacy in *Sicily*, was called *all-heal*. The plant

* Ibid.

F 4 *alyffum*,

alyſſum, or *madwort*, *garlic*, *agrimony*, and *oxy-
lapathum*, *ſharp-pointed dock*, were alſo highly
recommended. The effect of the *ſpongia cynorrhodi* is attributed to the great number of
inſects in that excreſcence ; whence, from its
animal ſalts, it is deemed a diuretic : and, for
this reaſon, Doctor MEAD ſays *, that the
learned BACCIUS, upon the authority of RHA-
ZES and JOANNES DAMASCENUS, recommends *cantharides* infuſed in butter-milk, and
made up into troches with flowers of *lentils*
and wine ; and Doctor KRAMER † boils ten
grains of the fine powder of *cantharides* in an
ounce and half or two ounces of the beſt *vinegar*, which is given warm to the patient in
the *hydrophobia*. Whether this preparation
deſtroys the troubleſome, nay dangerous effects of the *cantharides*, I will not take upon
me to determine ; but as theſe inſects abound
with acrid diuretic ſalts, it is probable, they
will produce, at leaſt increaſe, the *priapiſms*,
the known conſequences of *cantharides*, whether applied in bliſters, or given internally in
any form. The ſmalleſt bliſter will produce
a ſtrangury, in hot and bilious conſtitutions,
notwithſtanding it ſhould be armed with muſ-
lin, or well rubbed with *camphor* ; and even
half a grain of *cantharides*, powdered, has
brought on a ſtrong *ſatyriaſis*, or *furor uterinus*,

* MEAD's Eſſays on poiſons, p. 161.
† Commerc. *Norimberg*.

when

when given to youthful and vigorous perſons of a warm conſtitution.

The *pulvis antilyſſus*, firſt recommended by Mr. GEORGE DAMPIER, and communicated by Mr. SOUTHWELL to SIR HANS SLOANE, was publiſhed in the Philoſophical Tranſactions *; wherein SIR HANS SLOANE deſcribes the plant to be not the *Jews-ear*, but the *lichen* † : and in 1721 Doctor MEAD deſired this powder ſhould be inſerted in the *Pharmacopœia Londinenſis*.

Whatever ſucceſs may have attended the *pulvis antilyſſus*, it is certainly a powerful diuretic, and profeſſedly ordered by Doctor MEAD with that intention, as a preſervative againſt the progreſs of the poiſonous *saliva* of a mad dog. Doctor MEAD was too well acquainted with the uncertainty of this climate, not to be convinced, that, of all the ſecretions by which the ſaline particles of the poiſonous *saliva* could be diſcharged, there was none ſo likely to be obſtructed as perſpiration: and knowing, that, next to the diſcharge through the pores of the ſkin, the kidneys carry off the greateſt quantity of lymph, and ſupply the want of perſpiration; it was very conſiſtent, in that great phyſician, to direct a remedy which he knew acted as a powerful diuretic. But it has been queſtioned, by ſome

* Philoſophical Tranſactions, N° 237.
† See a deſcription of this plant taken from Mr. RAY, in Doctor MEAD's Eſſays on poiſons, p. 166.

expe-

experienced phyſicians, profeſſor BOERHAAVE, Baron VAN SWIETEN, and our accurate and ingenious botaniſt Doctor WATSON *, whether the *lichen cinereus terreſtris,* or *aſh-colored ground liverwort,* is endued with that quality which Doctor MEAD attributes to it. From the Doctor's examination of this moſſy plant ſo claſſed by profeſſor DILLENIUS, the ſeveral portions of acid water, oil, and coal, containing fixt ſalt which were produced, by diſtillation, will determine the queſtion, Whether it be a diuretic, or not? and ſuppoſe this plant not to have all the deſired efficacy, the other ingredient in the preſcription will eaſily be ſhewn to be ſufficient, of itſelf, to have anſwered the intended purpoſe. In the original receipt, in Mr. DAMPIER's family, the proportions of the *liverwort* and *black pepper* were equal; but Doctor MEAD reduced the quantity of pepper to only one third of the whole, left the pepper ſhould be too hot. Whoever will inquire into the opinion of the ancients, may take the following extract from that great naturaliſt Lord BACON †. " Pepper, ſays he, " by ſome of the ancients is noted to move " urine, when given in great quantity; which, " being given in ſmall quantity, moveth wind " in the ſtomach and guts, and ſo expelleth " by ſtool. But being in greater quantity, " diſſipateth the wind, and itſelf getteth to

---

* Philoſophical Tranſactions, vol. l. part ii. p. 681.
† BACON's Sylva Sylvarum, cent. i. v. 44.

" the

" the mefentery veins, and fo to the liver and
" reins; where, by heating and opening, it
" fendeth down urine more plentifully."

Thus it appears, that pepper was, many
years ago, acknowleged to be a diuretic; and
therefore the *pulvis antilyffus* may have an-
fwered Doctor MEAD's intentions, in many
cafes, although it was never looked upon, by
that excellent phyfician, as an infallible remedy, any more than any other medicine.
He well knew, it would not fucceed in fuch
cafes where it might heat too much: he pur-
pofely, therefore, leffened the quantity, to prevent heating, and gave it in warm milk, that
it might fheathe and leffen the acrimony of the
faliva, carry the powder more eafily through
the firft paffages, and fo into the blood. Dioscorides * and PALMARIUS recommend
the ufe of milk in all cafes of poifons: and as
in the difeafe arifing from the bite of a mad
dog, the bile is vifibly affected, the acefcent
quality of the milk renders it the more ufeful
to correct the acrimony of the bilious falts.
Doctor MEAD never imagined the *pulvis antilyffus* could be of ufe when the *hydrophobia* was
once come on: it is therefore plain, that, after
bleeding, he directed this powder as a preventive cure, to difcharge the acrid falts by
urine, which cold bathing would alfo affift.

* DIOSCORIDES De victus ratione demorforum a cane
rubiofo in theriaca, cap. ii. PALMARIUS loc. cit.

IV. The

IV. The poifonous effects of the *faliva* of a mad dog have very ftrenuoufly been afferted, by Doctor DESAULT *, to arife from worms contained in the *faliva* of the dog, and propagated in whatever creature it be inoculated; but the dormant ftate in which this *virus* hath lain many years, before it hath broken out, is a fufficient argument to overthrow that *hypothefis*, however fupported by the authority of BONETUS, ETMULLER, AVICENNA, and others. With a view of deftroying thofe infects, he adopts and recommends the boafted powder prefcribed by PALMARIUS, confifting of bitter and *vermifuge* herbs; to which Doctor DESAULT adds the *coralline*. PALMARIUS's† powder confifts of, the leaves of *rue, vervain,* the *leffer fage, plantain, polypody, common wormwood, mint, mugwort, baftard baum, (meliffophylon,) betony, St. John's wort,* and the *leffer centaury,* of each equal weight. Thefe are to be dried, and powdered, and half a drachm of the powder is to be taken upon an empty ftomach, and three hours before meals either with twice the quantity of fugar, or in wine, cyder, broth; or with honey, or butter, in the confiftence of an electary.

However ineffectual this prefcription muft appear, to every one who confiders the cafe

---

* DESAULT Differtation fur la rage, article ii.
† PALMARIUS, p. 344.

for which it was intended *, yet the fame intention has produced one of the moſt ſalutary
effects that mankind could receive, by ſug-
geſting to Doctor Desault a far more eaſy,
and more certain preventive cure. He ſays,
that from ſeeing worms of various kinds, and
almoſt all ſorts of verminous inſects, and cutaneous eruptions, deſtroyed by *mercury*, he
was induced to try what a mercurial unction
would do.

This method of preventing the ill conſequences of the bite of a mad dog, by a mercurial friction, was attended with all the favorable ſucceſs, Monſieur Desault, the firſt
inventor of it, could deſire; and has ſince, by
repeated cures, both in *Europe* and *Aſia*, confirmed the utility of this practice.

His method is, to rub upon the wound,
and all over the adjacent parts, one or two
drams of an ointment made of, *one third
part of mercury revived from cinnabar, one
third part of human fat, and as much of hog's
lard.*

The frictions are repeated every other day,
in the beginning; after the third time, every
third day; after the ſixth, every fourth, till
two or three ounces of the ointment be uſed;
always proportioning the quantity to the
ſtrength, age, conſtitution, ſex of the patient, and the ſtate of the bite.

---

* See the note at p. 16, of this Eſſay.

But

But fhould the patient have applied, many days after the bite; he then orders the frictions to be daily repeated every day, for four or five days.

Doctor DESAULT very fenfibly adds *, that fhould the *mercury* occafion a flight falivation, it could not but be attended with good fuc-cefs: for, fays he, the poifon of the *rabies*, fticking to the *faliva*, and *mercury* naturally taking its courfe towards the mouth, can it be doubted that this fovereign antidote, in many diforders, fhould not alfo deftroy that which occafions the *hydrophobia?*

Common experience teftifies, that, in the cure of venereal complaints, where *mercury* is applied, and a falivation is to be prevented, emollient clyfters, or the mildeft laxative and diuretic purges, turn the courfe of the hu-mors, and prevent the ufual effect of the *mer-cury* upon the falival glands; fo that, in this prefent cafe, where the tainted *faliva* is to be difcharged, a falivation may be either encou-raged, or checked, as the practitioner thinks moft expedient.

Doctor DESAULT makes no alteration in the perfon's food, or meals, provided he avoids all excefs. He allows the moderate ufe of wine, to raife the patient's courage; and ftrongly re-commends, that, far from leaving the perfon alone, he fhould be conftantly in chearful company; who, however, muft be careful ne-

* DESAULT Differtation fur la rage, p. 305.

ver

ver to let their difcourfe turn on fuch fubjects as have any relation to the patient's cafe.

The late Mr. JOHN DOUGLAS, a furgeon of great abilities, publifhed in 1738, on a fingle half fheet of paper *, his recommendation of the mercurial friction, for this very difeafe. He directs one dram of a mercurial ointment, confifting of

One pound of pure quickfilver, and the fame quantity of human fat, and of hog's lard, and two ounces of clarified turpentine, mixed according to art,

to be rubbed into the wounds, and parts adjacent; and Doctor MEAD's *pulvis antilyffus* to be taken every morning in a glafs of wine and water, water, or cow's milk warm. The unction is to be repeated every evening, and the powder every morning fafting, during three weeks, leaving off the unction two or three days when the mouth begins to be fore, to prevent a falivation. Then the *mercury* is to be purged off, and in about three weeks or a month after, when the patient has recruited, he is to ufe the cold bath.

It is plain, from thefe directions, that Mr. DOUGLAS's intentions were to difcharge

---

* A fure method of preventing, and the moft probable way of curing, the *hydrophobia*, i. e. the dread of water, after the bite of a mad dog; a difeafe hitherto found incurable by the practitioners of all nations. By JOHN DOUGLAS, Surgeon, and F. R. S. *February* 26, 1738. Given *gratis* in *Lad-lane* near *Guildhall.*

the

the poifonous *faliva*, by the falival glands, by perfpiration, and by the urinary paffages. Where the *hydrophobia* is come on, he advifes plentiful bleeding, and the rubbing in a large quantity of the ointment into the *axillary* and *inguinal* glands, and all over the limbs.

To thefe intentions of difcharging the poifonous *faliva* of the mad dog, through the falival glands, the pores of the fkin, and the urinary paffages, by *mercurial* applications, Monfieur Du Choisel's method is to be fubjoined, as more efficacious in the climate he lives in.

In thofe hotter climates, the mercurial ointment is ufed with equal fuccefs. Monfieur Du Choisel *, apothecary to the *Jefuit* miffion at *Pondicherry*, in the *Eaft Indies*, makes an ointment of

One ounce of crude mercury, extinguifhed in two drams of turpentine; of mutton fuet three ounces.

The heat of the climate determines Mr. Du Choisel to prefer *mutton fuet* to *hog's lard*. He rubs in one dram upon the wounded part, keeping the wound open as much as poffible; the next day he repeats the unction on all the bitten member, and purges the patient with a dram of his mercurial pills; the third day

---

* Du Choisel's method of treating perfons bit by mad animals, p. 17.

he

he rubs the ointment only over the bitten part, he gives a fmall mercurial bolus, or the fourth part of the mercurial pills above mentioned. Thus he continues for ten days to rub in a dram of the ointment every morning, and to give the laxative bolus, which commonly procures the patient two or three ftools, and hinders the mercury from affecting the upper parts. At the end of ten days, he purges again, with the fame pills, and difmiffes the patient.

The mercurial pills are compofed of

Three drams of crude mercury, extinguifhed in one dram of turpentine; of the beft rhubarb, colloquintida in powder, and gutta gamba, of each two drams. The whole to be made up, with a fufficient quantity of clarified honey. The dofe one dram.

This method is only adapted to fuch perfons who apply to Mr. Du CHOISEL, immediately after being bitten. After two or three weeks, the difeafe having taken a deeper root, Mr. Du CHOISEL increafes the dofe of the medicines, and continues them for a longer time. The dofe is alfo proportioned to the age and conftitution of children, a fmall quantity of the ointment is rubbed in for fifteen days, and he purges them, once in three days, with fyrup of *rhubarb*. As to regimen, Mr. Du CHOISEL forbids his patients the ufe

G of

of things tart or acid, of all crude meats, and
such as are hard to digeft.

Thus it is obvious, from Mr. Du Choisel's account, that crude *mercury* expels the
poifonous *faliva* through the falival glands;
and that, to prevent an obftruction in thofe
glands, it is neceffary, in the *Eaft Indies*, to
purge with the above mentioned pills.   But
what gives the greateft fatisfaction, is the cafe
he relates *, of a woman who had the *hydro-*
phobia, and was cured by rubbing in three
drams of the mercurial ointment, at a time,
and fo repeated, night and morning, till a
plentiful falivation came on; which relieved
her head, removed the *hydrophobia*, and cured
her entirely; the falivation being carried off
by a *dyfenteric* purging, which was alfo remedied by means of a laxative electary, with
rhubarb, taken in the morning, and a dofe of
diafcordium at night.

This ferves to prove the efficacy of *mer-*
cury in this difeafe, as well as in the *lues ve-*
nerea.   And certainly *mercury* in a crude ftate,
purified, and cleanfed, has this peculiar advantage attending it, well known to thofe who
adminifter it frequently, that it neither irritates, nor is fo uncertain in it's operation, as
moft mercurial preparations are; for which
reafon it is fafely applied externally, and may

* P. 25, 26.

be

be given internally, in a ſtate of inflammation, in this diſeaſe, as well as in the venereal one. Experience demonſtrates the ſucceſs of crude *mercury*, in Monſieur Du Choisel's curing above 300 patients, from the year
1749 to 1753.

In *Aſia*, and *Europe*, mercurials have been
given internally, to prevent the bad effects
ariſing from the bite of a mad dog; and I
ſhould have mentioned them, according to the
time of their being introduced into practice,
before Meſſieurs Douglas and Du Choisel's
methods, had not theſe two practitioners followed the ſame intentions with Doctor Desault; and therefore it was proper to place
them in that order.

In *Aſia*, where the heat of the climate produces a profuſe perſpiration, and the inhabitants require a ſupply of animal particles, and
of ſpirituous liquors, the *Chineſe* make uſe of
the following medicine; which, from it's
great ſucceſs, was brought over to *England* by
Sir George Cobb, and Lady Frederick,
in hopes it might prove as effectual in *Europe*,
as in the *Eaſt Indies*, for the cure of the diſtemper ariſing from the bite of a mad dog.

The preſcription is as follows:

*Take of native and factitious cinnabar, of
each twenty-four grains; of muſk, ſixteen
grains: Let them be powdered, and well mixed
together.*

A

As soon as poffible, after the perfon is bitten, he is to take this powder in a glafs or teacup full of *arrack*. If no fymptom appears, this dofe is thought to fecure the patient, for thirty days; but if the leaft fymptom is upon him, then the dofe is to be repeated three hours after.

From the compofition of factitious *cinnabar*, and the chymical analyfis of native *cinnabar*, it appears, that they are both compofed of *mercury*, and *fulphur*, the firft in a proportion of above three to one, and the latter of fix to one of *mercury* to the *fulphur*. The other ingredient *mufk*, is an animal fubftance, which promotes a gentle fweat, without heating, raifes the fpirits, eafes pain, and ufually brings on a refrefhing fleep. It is known to be an excellent antifpafmodic; and Doctor WALL, has recorded in the Philofophical Tranfactions *, it's good effects in convulfive diforders, particularly in two perfons attended with *fubfultus tendinum*, extreme anxiety, and want of fleep, from the bite of a mad dog. Doctor HUXHAM fays †, that *mufk* has a great power of expelling the morbid humors through the pores of the fkin, without heating too much. And Mr. PRINGLE ‖ has given fixteen grains of *mufk*, with twenty-five grains of *native cinnabar*, and as many of *cinnabar*

---

* Philofophical Tranfactions, Nᵒ 474.
† HUXHAM De aere & morbis, tom. ii. p. 125.
‖ Phyfical Effays, vol. ii. p. 252.

of antimony, in a glafs of brandy, to a lady, in a bad fit of the gout. Doctor HILL, in his *Materia Medica**, alfo commends *mufk* as a cordial and antihyfteric.

This prefcription, then, is not only of ufe to the *Chinefe*, as a diaphoretic, antifpafmodic, and antihyfteric ; but may be of great fervice, alfo, in *Europe*, efpecially among thofe who have no diflike to perfumes, or feed much upon animal food, and delight in fpices, and high feafonings : but, notwithftanding I readily acknowlege the good effects of *mufk*, in fpafmodic, epileptic, and hyfteric cafes ; yet I muft fairly own, that, in putrid difeafes, where the *crafis* of the blood has been broken, and the *vis vitæ* much impaired, *mufk* has failed me, in fuch conftitutions as have been accuftomed to a vegetable diet, and very little animal food : and when neither the *mufk julep*, nor *mufk* in fubftance, would take place, the *camphorated julep*, with acids, has fucceeded. This doth not quite invalidate the ufe of the *mufk* and *cinnabar*, in the cafe of a bite from a mad dog ; it may certainly fucceed, even in our climate, as a preventive, but whenever the difeafe attains any degree of putridity, it will not be fafe, entirely to rely upon it.

Doctor JAMES is the firft practitioner, in *Europe*, who has advifed a mercurial medicine to be taken internally, for the prevention and

---

* HILL's Materia Medica, p. 861.

cure

cure of this terrible difeafe. It appears, from his publications, that, towards the end of the year 1731, the Doctor recommended the ufe of *turpeth mineral,* or *mercurius emeticus flavus,* with the fame intentions as this medicine is given in the venereal diftemper; and from the fuccefs of it in which, he moft probably took the hint.

In a pamphlet, printed in 1741, he writes to profeffor BOERHAAVE, that the following prefcription had, in *February* 1732, cured two foxhounds, actually mad, and to whom neither dipping in falt water, nor the *tin* medicines, had done any good. He gave from feven and twelve grains, to twenty-four, of the *turpeth mineral,* to one dog, who had a plentiful falivation, and recovered.

As a prefervative, Doctor JAMES prefcribed to perfons bitten, as follows:

Take of turpeth mineral twelve grains, of compound powder of contrayerva one dram, of Venice treacle as much as is requifite to make three boluffes; one to be taken every night, with an antihyfteric julep.

This method was attended with fuccefs in the cure of a young man of eighteen, another of feventeen, and a girl of fourteen years of age, who were all bitten by dogs who proved mad; but not one of thofe perfons had the leaft fign of an *hydrophobia,* nor any other aggravating fymptoms, than dejection, and tremors.

mors. It does not appear that any external application was made to them, although the Doctor in this pamphlet, and in the succeeding edition in 1743, directs the use of Doctor DESAULT's mercurial ointment, and also the *pulvis antilyssus*, and *cinnabarine* powder.

In autumn 1760, Doctor JAMES published a loose half-sheet, of *Instructions for preventing and curing of canine madness*; in which, having labored much to prove himself the first inventor of the mercurial method, at least taken internally, which there seems no reason to dispute, although Doctor JAMES owns that Doctor DESAULT was the first that made use of the mercurial ointment, as Mr. DOUGLAS informed him; the Doctor proceeds to recommend the rubbing in of a dram of a mercurial ointment every day, during a week, and even twice a day, without raising a salivation. He also advises the *turpeth mineral*, but in less quantities, and with a different intention. The prescription is altered thus:

Take of turpeth mineral from three to eight grains, according to the strength of the patient, and the degree of infection received; camphire an equal quantity, to be made with conserve of hips into a bole. To be taken three times, alternately, every other night.

Doctor JAMES's intentions plainly appear, first, by his direction of the *turpeth mineral*,

G 4

the

the *compound powder of contrayerva*, and the
Venice treacle, to have vomited and pro-
moted both the falivary and cuticular difcharges; but finding the irritation of the
mercurial vomit too great to allow of the
other ingredients to operate, he changes his
defign, and mixes equal quantities of *turpeth mineral* and *camphor*, to promote perfpiration, and hinder the *turpeth*, as he fays,
from vomiting; but the *naufea* caufed frequently by the *camphor*, will, probably, dif-
appoint the intended effect; efpecially when
the ftomach is in a ftate of irritation, from
the vitiated *faliva* admitted into it: fo that
even this mixture, long fince recommended
by medical authors, to fheathe the acrid
particles of mercurial preparations, and to
promote their operation, as alterants and dia-
phoretics, in venereal cafes, cannot be fo
well adapted, in the cafe of perfons really
bitten by mad dogs. The *turpeth mineral*
can therefore only be given, with fafety, at
fuch an age, and in fuch conftitutions as are
of a relaxed texture, leucophlegmatic, or
debilitated; in which, as in many venereal
inftances, the folids and fluids require a degree of irritation, to enable them to perform
their functions and fecretions: but where
there is already a tenfion, which is likely to
be increafed, and produce fpafms, a milder
method of introducing mercury is to be
pre-

preferred, which, even in the higheſt degree of inflammation, owing to an acrid venereal *virus*, is known to have had all the deſired effect, without cauſing the leaſt pain, heat, or ſenſible inconveniency. And this is the introduction of crude mercury into the blood, by means of a mercurial ointment.

In the conſideration of the following caſes I ſhall endeavor to make it appear what kind of treatment, and medicines, have proved chiefly beneficial.

SECTION

SECTION IV.

OBSERVATIONS.

CASE I.

A NARRATIVE *of an uncommon* CASE, *which happened about* 25 *years ago, in the neighbourhood of* Salisbury, *from the bite of a mad dog. Communicated by Doctor* HELE, *physician at* Salisbury.

A Young lady, about twenty years of age, and of a good healthy constitution, feeding her little favorite dog, at dinner, was bitten by the finger, so that it bled a little, on both sides, where his teeth had broke the skin; and she unfortunately sucked the blood, and spit it out. The dog had been sullen and sleepy all that day, and refused his victuals. The next day the gamekeeper, suspecting madness, confined him, and in two days he died.

The young lady, alarmed at this terrible accident, came the next day to me for advice. I ordered her to lose eight ounces of blood, from the arm, to take Doctor MEAD's *pulvis antilyssus* for six mornings, and, after that, to undergo the usual immersions in the sea,

drinking

drinking half a pint of the fame water, every morning, for a month. She obferved the former part of thefe directions, and then repaired to *Southampton*, for the benefit of the fea water. The next day after her arrival, fhe was dipped; but being kept under water for fome time, and then dipped again, and again, with very fhort intervals, fhe was fo much frightened, that fhe could not be prevailed upon to bathe a fecond time, or fo much as to drink the water; but fhe refided there the whole month (the time allotted for this courfe), and then returned to her friends, concealing from them the inexcufable omiffions fhe had been guilty of: and they had not the leaft diftruft but fhe had regularly conformed to the whole courfe prefcribed.

She continued quite well, for five months, and about the expiration of that time fhe was feized fuddenly with a chill, foon after fhe had fat down to make tea for the company who had dined there that day; and this little *rigor* was immediately fucceeded by fo total a *fyncope*, that fhe fell from her chair, and remained fpeechlefs and fenfelefs on the floor, for fome minutes. She was carried up ftairs, and foon put to bed, and fome time after, fhe grew warm, and fhe had reachings to vomit. She took two ounces of *ipecacuanha* wine, with half a dram of *fpir. lavendul. comp.* which had good effect, by relieving the great load and oppreffion on the ftomach, and promoting a

per-

perspiration, which kept her easy a good part of the following night: but in the morning I found her low, hot, and restless, with a quick weak pulse, and complaining of great weight, and uneasiness about the *præcordia*, with a *subsultus tendinum*, and frequent twitchings, and startings. Blisters were immediately applied to the back and arms, and sinapisms to the feet, and the diaphoretic medicines exhibited as usual in such cases. Every thing went on much the same that night; and finding the patient not at all relieved the next morning, but growing rather *comatose* and delirious, with the same low quick pulse, I ordered blisters to be applied to the head and thighs. The next morning I found her relieved of the *coma*, and *delirium*, but the *subsultus tendinum*, and convulsive twitchings, much the same; and the nurse told me, that she often, in the night, called for liquor, but could not drink it when brought to her. I never had, till then, the least thought of the bite of the mad dog; but now, being apprehensive that this symptom was somewhat of the *hydrophobous* kind, I asked her whether she would drink a draught of any of the liquors appointed for her common drink. She expressed great desire of drinking, but said, the liquors offered her by the nurse went against her stomach. I asked her what she herself would chuse to drink. She thought, that if she could be indulged with some *Rhenish* wine and water, it would

be

be the moſt agreeable draught ſhe ever had in
her life. Both were ſoon brought, and I my-
ſelf mixed them, by the bed-ſide, that ſhe
might not ſuſpect that we had, in any ſhape,
deceived her. She caught at the glaſs, with
great eagernefs, but the moment it touched
her lips, ſhe puſhed it from her, and, as I
preſſed it to her mouth, with ſome little force,
ſhe as ſtrenuouſly puſhed it away, and, with a
ſmall ſtruggle, fell into a ſtrong convulſion,
which laſted ſome time, and ſeemed to be attended with the ſame ſort of fulneſs of the
throat, and ſtrangulation, as frequently accom-
pany hyſteric diſorders. I then pronounced the
whole illneſs to be the effect of the dog's bite,
and that this averſion to drinking was the
worſt ſymptom that could befal us. I ordered her a bolus with *cinnabar. antimon. pulv.
ad guttetam,* $\overline{aa}$ ℈j, to be given every ſix hours,
which ſhe ſwallowed tolerably well, but not a
drop of liquid could be got into the mouth,
even by force, without cauſing a return of the
convulſive fits. The next morning, I ordered
a bliſter to be applied all round the neck, as
broad as her neck (which was naturally pretty
long) would admit of, and the bolus to be repeated as before. The next day ſhe would
take down a little quantity of warmed liquid
at a time, though it often ſeemed to put her
into great agonies. After this manner, in
ſhort, we kept on, with the addition of five
grains of *ſal. volatil. ammoniac.* to each bolus ;
the

the exhibition of glyfters occafionally, and fuch other few difcretionary alterations or additions, for ten days longer; when, after a gentle *diaphorefis*, for almoft three days and three nights, the fever, and every concomitant bad fymptom, entirely left her, and fhe got ftrength apace, flept found and quiet fleeps at night, fat up for feveral hours at a time every day, and converfed very agreeably and fedately with any of the family who vifited her.

Thus fhe went on for a fortnight, or longer, and then, one morning, after fhe had been up about an hour, and was talking, in a pleafant manner, with a young lady of her intimate acquaintance, fhe fell into a phrenzy, and, in lefs than an hour, feemed quite a maniac.

The pulfe was very quick, and, though not full, yet fhe was blooded by force, a glyfter given, and a large blifter applied to the back part of the head, and all this time fhe attempted to bite every body that came near her, which fhe was never once inclined to do, in all her former fever. In this raving condition fhe continued for thirty hours, when fhe fell afleep, with the great fatigue, foon got into a profufe fweat, and became quite fenfible again.

It is to be obferved, that this paroxyfm of phrenzy began about twenty-four hours before the new moon; and although it left her in the manner above mentioned, and fhe continued, apparently, as well as ever fhe was in

her

her life, for the fpace of three weeks, and upwards; yet, about thirty hours before the next
new moon, the fever and phrenzy returned,
with the fame violence as before, but continued not above twelve hours, when it went
off with the ufual fleep, and fweat: and thus,
for the fpace of five months longer, we had
the raving paroxyfms, and clear intermiffions,
more or lefs, about the time of the new
moon: but every month the raving fits fhort-
ned, and the laft of all held not above half an
hour; when fhe voluntarily threw herfelf on
the bed, and flept and fweat as before.

During the whole time, the large blifter on
the *occiput* was kept open, the *cinnabar* bolus
given twice in twenty-four hours, and gentle
cordial purgatives were adminiftred, as occafion
required. The *catamenia* were regular, before,
at, and after the whole courfe of the diforder.
She purfued the fame method for fome
months longer, the blifter ftill kept open the
whole time, as large as all the hinder part of
the head would admit, and fhe had never
afterwards the leaft fymptom of any relapfe,
though fhe married about a year after, and had
feveral children, and died about nine years after
her recovery.

It is further to be obferved, in the firft place,
That even the fmall preventive courfe fhe followed, may have protracted the appearance of
any bad fymptom for fome months, and might
likewife be the principal caufe of their remark-

able deviation from the common courfe of fuch fevers, when they did come on.

Secondly, I think it is to be confidered, how far the blifter, round the neck, might alter the quality of the *faliva*, remove that refemblance of a *hydrophobia*, and avail in reftoring a power of deglutition, though with fome difficulty.

And, Thirdly, I would beg leave to mention the power and efficacy, I have frequently experienced, of *cinnabarine* medicines (without *mufk*), but joined with *pulvis ad guttetam*, in convulfions of almoft all kinds, either with or without fever; and that, whenever I have added the *valerian* root, inftead of the *pulvis ad guttetam*, it has generally ftimulated too much, and increafed, rather than diminifhed, the convulfive fymptoms.

November 14,
  1760.   H. HELE.

REMARKS.

This cafe is the ftrongeft proof of the validity of Doctor MEAD's opinion, in favor of a nervous fluid, and of this fluid being particularly affected by the vitiated *faliva* of the mad dog: for it feems, without any previous or immediate effect on any of the blood-veffels, or on any of the tendons, or large nerves, to have been abforbed by the lymphatic veffels, .

and

and to have circulated through the whole mafs of fluids.

The bleeding, and diuretic *pulvis antilyssus*, may, as Doctor HELE obferves, have delayed the fatal effects fome months; but the fingle immerfion in fea water was of no advantage; fince it only ferved to terrify the young lady to that degree, that fhe could not bear the thoughts of repeating the bathing.

No pain in the finger which had been bitten, and healed, without any particular care, in two or three days; no pricking, fhooting, or darting pain up the arm, came on, to fhew any particular irritation of the nerves externally. But at the end of five months, when near the full moon, a fudden chillnefs and *syncope* feized her, followed by reachings to vomit, oppreffion of the *præcordia*, attended with anxiety, a quick pulfe, *fubfultus tendinum*, and frequent catchings. Can it be doubted, that the nervous fluid and the whole mafs of blood were wholly affected, and that this was an effort of nature to expel the poifon? Nay, more; if it be confidered, that, three days after, the *hydrophobia*, and *naufea* at the ftomach, came on: is not this the critical difcharge by which the acrimonious falts of the *faliva* were to be thrown off? and did not the blifter, applied round the neck, and continued a long while open, ferve to draw off, as in the *angina*, part of the humor from the falival glands, and, of courfe, leffen the degree of irritation

H all

all along the *œsophagus*, which caused the
hydrophobia?

Ten days after this seizure, a *diaphoresis*
broke out, which lasted three days, and three
nights; and this sweating carried off the fever, and other symptoms. The *cinnabar* and
pulvis ad guttetam, with the addition of *sal.
ammoniacum*, produced this effect in the blood,
and no extraordinary motion was found in it;
during a fortnight after, her mind recovering
also its serenity and chearfulness.—But, about
twenty-four hours before the next full moon,
suddenly a phrenzy comes on, and the young
lady becomes a perfect *maniac*, in less than an
hour. She is furious, endeavors to bite, and,
by means of a profuse sweat, she recovers her
senses. The symptoms return about thirty
hours before the next full moon, last not so
long a while, but every month, repeatedly
five times, Doctor HELE saw them, and con-
quered them, at last, by a perseverance in the
use of the *cinnabar* powder, and keeping a
blister perpetually open on the back of the
head.

Can there be stronger proofs of a nervous
fluid particularly affected in this stage of the
disease? Does not the power of the moon
shew itself in those periodical returns? Does
the least sign of inflammation now appear by
the blood, and is it not owing to the seafon-
able evacuations, and, indeed, to Doctor HELE's
whole prudent directions? Does not this

young

young lady's case set Doctor MEAD's opinion beyond all dispute?

I cannot pass over one very necessary observation; that, in the whole course of this disorder, the *menses* appeared regularly: therefore the blood had, all along, a due fluidity, agreeable to what professor BOERHAAVE, and other authors, have observed *.

CASE II.

THE CASE of ELIZABETH BRYANT, published by Doctor NUGENT, deserves notice: and I have extracted it from the Doctor's Essay, in order to make some remarks upon it.

ELIZABETH BRYANT, twenty-two years of age, healthy, and of a good habit of body, chiefly sanguine, and phlegmatic, was, on the 23d of *June*, 1757, bit, by a mad turnspit dog, on the third finger of her right hand, which bled some few drops; and on the back of the hand, the skin of which was pinched through, but did not bleed. The sores healed soon, without any particular application; the dog died the next day. Upon her being restless and fretful, Mr. WRIGHT, a surgeon of reputation, ordered her to the sea, where she was dipped, till she could bear it no longer.

* Cruorem valde liquidum, & vix in aëre concrescentem. BOERHAAVII Aphorism. 1140.

On

On her return he bled her in the arm, and gave her four doses of Doctor Mead's *pulvis anti-lyffus*. On the 20th of *July* she was put into the cold bath, which treatment was repeated four mornings fucceflively; then, upon complaining of a numbnefs and pain in the arm and fhoulder of the hand that was bitten, Sir George Cobb's medicine, of *cinnabar* and *mufk*, was given. She thought her fpirits greatly relieved, and faid fhe was very well. The appearance of the *catamenia* prevented her ufing the cold bath next day. On the 27th of *July*, in the morning, about five hours before the full moon, fhe was, *all at once*, feized with a pain in the middle finger, and at the back of the hand, where fhe had been bitten, darting up her arm and fhoulder, acrofs her throat, and then fhe was afraid of being choaked; and ufed to lay hold of her throat as if to prevent it's clofing up; could not bear the fight of water, nor hear even the noife of falling water, which, as alfo the barking and howling of dogs, brought on the pain to an intolerable degree, attended with a *fuffocation, fhort breathing, dizzinefs, rifings at her ftomach, breaft, and throat*, and ftrong catchings, as if fhe was going into convulfions. In this ftate Doctor Nugent vifited her; and, by prefenting a bafon of water, was confirmed that Elizabeth Bryant was feized with an *hydrophobia*. She had immediately fifteen ounces of blood drawn, and a paper

paper of the *cinnabarine* powder was ordered to be taken every three hours, in honey; a pill, of two grains of the *extractum thebaicum,* every three hours, with the powders, till reft could be procured; and a plaifter of *galbanum,* with half an ounce of the fame *extractum thebaicum,* to be applied to the throat and neck. In the evening fhe was eafier, and could recollect fhe had been blooded, and with great difficulty fwallowed fome broth. Her blood looked very well. The powders and *opium* pill were repeated every three hours, and the wounded arm rubbed with warm fallad oil, feveral times a day. The 28th of *July* fhe was bled again, to twenty ounces, and had a clyfter of *antimonial* wine, the pills and powders repeated, and the fallad oil rubbed as before. She could fwallow liquids better; was ordered ten grains of *turpeth mineral,* and another clyfter. *Monday* morning, the 29th, fhe loft twelve ounces of blood, the powders continued, was directed to drink often of barley water with *nitre* and the *galbanum* plaifter renewed. In the evening every way better, the pain in her arm and hand quite gone, but her fear of dogs and water remain. The *mufk* and *cinnabar* to be taken as before, the oil to be rubbed in, and only two grains of the *extract* of *opium* to be given at night. *Tuefday,* 30th *July,* fhe was fick at her ftomach, fweat much in the night, complained of pains, owing, it was thought, to cold contracted. The clyfter,

fter, the powders every fix hours, and the fallad oil, were repeated. The *nitre* was omitted, and the *opium* quite laid afide. She
fweat much this day, and drank plentifully of
water-gruel and baum tea. The clyfter
worked well. *Wednefday* morning, 31ft, the
pains were gone. She had been fick at mid-
night, after which fhe had fweat profufely;
all fymptoms difappeared, except her dread of
water and dogs. The *opium* plaifter was removed, and the powders continued every fix
hours, but in the evening were only ordered
night and morning. On *Thurfday* the fymptoms returned, but abated after her drinking
tea. This night fhe was much frighted by
dreams. On *Friday* morning a clyfter was
given; the dread of water was now quite
over, only it made her giddy. *Sunday* fhe
mended in appetite, ftrength, and fpirits, and
continued fo till the 16th of *Auguft*, when the
young woman, through the folly or wicked-
nefs of a man and woman, was thrown into
the greateft terrors. An opiate was given
that night, and the *cinnabar* powders were
directed in *elder flower* tea. She was vomited
with *ipecacuanha* wine, bled to about twelve
ounces, and took faline draughts with bitter
and antihyfteric medicines. Doctor NUGENT
judging the cafe to be now hyfterical, directed
the following powder, which Doctor HAL-
LET, of *Exeter*, had ufed with great fuccefs.

℞ *Af.*

℞ *Af. fœtid.* gr. xij. *mofch.* gr. x. *camphor.*
gr. vj. *m. f. pulvis.*

This was given in the afternoon in a bolus,
and repeated at bed-time, with the faline
draughts between whiles. The next day,
after fweating confiderably, and fleeping well,
fhe was much mended, in all refpects. Two
faline draughts were ordered for the day, and
the fœtid bolus at night; and on the 4th of
September fhe was fo well, as to require no
more medicines, and has remained well ever
fince.

REMARKS.

This Cafe of ELIZABETH BRYANT plainly
fhews how greatly both the body and mind
are affected by this terrifying accident of the
bite of a mad dog. From the account, and
Doctor NUGENT's very ingenious and juft obfervations, it is evident, this young woman was
bitten by a dog in whom the heat of the wea-
ther in the month of *June,* the fituation the
animal was placed in, frequently as a turnfpit,
and perhaps the want of water, had raifed a
fever, and, as is common, a *delirium* enfued;
in which fit he bit ELIZABETH BRYANT:
but fhe was not apprized of his madnefs, till,
having offered him fome minced meat, he
could not fwallow it, frothed much at the
mouth, and flavered. His dying the next

day,

day, without violence, and a dog being killed raving mad, three weeks after, who had eaten the meat refufed and flavered on by the other; put it out of doubt, that the acute fever, raifed in the turnfpit dog, had fufficiently produced, before his death, that degree of acrimony in his *faliva*, as ftrongly to affect not only the other dog, but ELIZABETH BRYANT alfo.

From the affurances given her, by a neighbour, that the dog did not die mad, but choaked by fomething fticking in his throat, fhe feems to have had no further anxiety, till about three weeks after; when, probably, the madnefs of the other dog brought the accident frefh again into her mind. She then becomes of an unfettled temper, reftlefs, and fearful of dogs and water. Mr. WRIGHT attempts the ufual preventive cure, and, finding no effect from the fea-water bath, which fhe could bear no longer, he bled her, gave Doctor MEAD's *pulvis antilyffus*, and put her into the cold bath, which was left off on the appearance of the *menfes*.

This treatment, prudent and well intended, although it might protract the effects of the latent *virus*, yet it did not prevent it from fhewing itfelf: firft, by the appearance of two pimples, with white heads, on the back of the hand; and after, by a numbnefs and pain in the arm, hand, and fhoulder, of the bitten arm. Upon this, the *cinnabar* and *mufk* medicine being adminiftred, fhe found relief

from

from her pains, and her spirits were raised, for a while; but, five hours before the full moon, the pains from the bitten parts shoot regularly up the arm to her throat, and, as these advance, the terrors of her mind increase. Doctor NUGENT, in these circumstances, orders the young woman to be blooded; and, being chiefly of a sanguine constitution, the bleedings are repeated, during the course of the illness, till she had lost near sixty ounces of blood: and if these evacuations, together with the regular course of the *menses*, be attended to, there seems the same event to have followed, as in the person from whom Doctors HARTLEY and SANDYS drew 120 ounces *. The *cinnabar* medicine and *opium* are then directed, to promote sweat, assuage the pains, and relax the nervous system so as to remove the spasms, and the irritation which caused them; and also to quiet the mind, by procuring sleep.

Doctor NUGENT was so desirous of avoiding all kind of irritation, that he rejoices at his omission of the *turpeth mineral* bolus which he had prescribed; and even declares †, as a caution to others, that he should not have directed *antimonial* clysters, on account of their irritation, had not the free use of *opium* made their stimulating quality, as he thought, necessary.

---

* Philosophical Transactions, N° 448.
† NUGENT's Essay on the *hydrophobia*, p. 99, 100.

The

The Doctor tried to preferve his patient from too great a heat and inflammation, by the ufe of *nitre*, but this falt proved naufeous; and therefore he contented himfelf with diluting, by means of *water gruel* and *baum tea*. His directions proved fuccefsful; but the mind, like the body, remained weakened, and liable to a relapfe upon the firft furprize. The inadvertence or mifchievous defign of the perfons who affrighted her, threw her into all the former terrors, and fhe felt, as fhe thought, the fame pains; but a vomit feafonably given that night, to remove a loathing and ficknefs at the ftomach; her being blooded two days after, and the courfe of antihyfteric medicines, reftored that due ftate of the folids and fluids which conftitutes health; and, no doubt, proper encouragement, and comfort, alfo recovered her mind to it's former chearfulnefs and tranquillity.

Upon the whole, ELIZABETH BRYANT's cafe appears to be an acute, not a putrid one; and the neceffary evacuations, together with her fright, may have produced the high degree of *hyfterics* which followed.

CASE

CASE III, IV, and V.

THE 29th *December*, 1751, Mr. JOHN MEHEW, a farmer of *Godmanchefter* in the county of *Huntingdon*, having been abfent from home a few days, returned in the evening, and was informed that his yard dog was run mad, and had bitten eight cows, moft of them with calf, and two fows with pig; all which refufed to eat or drink, and died mad. The cows had the *pewter medicine* given them, by way of drench, feveral times, but without fuccefs.

This evening, *December* the 29th, one of the cows, being thought bitten, had been loofened, they having been all tied up, foon after they were bitten. She was no fooner at liberty, than fhe ran furioufly up and down the yard, endeavoring to do all the mifchief poffible, but was fecured by JOHN JONES, the man fervant, whom the cow bit in the fore finger, which was much torn. The fame evening Mr. MEHEW going to affift in giving the fame cow the drench of the *pewter medicine*, fhe bit him on the back of the left hand, and tore it much. The cow would not admit of the leaft drop of the drench, and flavered a great quantity into the bowl, in which, not knowing what had happened, Mrs. MEHEW dipped her fingers, and tafted

the

the liquor, to feel if it were not too hot. Being told the cow had flavered in it, fhe was much terrified.

Upon being fent for, I met the late Mr. HENRY HAWKINS, furgeon and apothecary at *Huntingdon*, who dreffed Mr. MEHEW's and JOHN JONES's wounds in the following manner. Firft, the wounds were cleared from the *faliva* with dry foft lint, then they were dilated, and fuffered to bleed, the blood being wafhed off with warm milk and water, and the wounds dried, they were dreffed with pledgits of lint dipped in warm *oil of turpentine*, over which, cataplafms of bread and milk, with *Venice treacle*, were applied. Mr. MEHEW, and his fervant JOHN JONES, were then blooded plentifully, and at night they and Mrs. MEHEW were vomited with *vinum ipecacuanhæ* and *oxymel fcilliticum*: after the operation, a cordial draught was given to each of them. The next morning they took Doctor MEAD's *pulvis antilyffus* in warm cow's milk. Mr. MEHEW's hand, and JOHN JONES's finger, were dreffed with pledgits fpread with *unguentum e gummi elemi*, after rubbing on the lips of the wounds, and over the back of Mr. MEHEW's hand, and JOHN JONES's finger, about one dram of the *unguentum cæruleum fortius*.

I directed them to take, each of them, two ounces of Doctor FULLER's *decoctum antilyffum*, in the afternoon at five o'clock. The

next

next day Mr. MEHEW and JOHN JONES were dreffed with the fame ointments, adding only to the *unguentum e gummi elemi* fome *mercurius præcipitatus ruber*, to keep the wounds open, and difcharging. The *pulvis antilyffus* and *decoctum antilyffum* were continued eight days, after which, the *Chinefe cinnabar* medicine was directed, with this difference, that Mrs. MEHEW took the powder with a julep made up with *pennyroyal* water, *rue* water, tincture of *caftor*, and of *valerian*, and fyrup of *faffron*; and Mr. MEHEW and his fervant JONES took it with a fpoonful of *rum* and water.

By this method no bad fymptom appeared, and the wounds were permitted to heal at the month's end, the mercurial ointment having always kept them free from inflammation. I advifed the ufe of the cold bath; but, fatisfied with their cure, they did not chufe to plunge into cold water in that fharp feafon of the year, in the midft of froft and fnow; and have never felt any bad confequence, either from their bites, or apprehenfions; being all alive, and in perfect health, at this time.

REMARKS.

That not only the dog was mad, but alfo the cattle whom he bit, is evident, from their all dying furious. That Mr. MEHEW and his fervant JONES received the *faliva* of the cow, with

with their wounds, I make not the leaft doubt
of. But although I am perſuaded of the
efficacy of mercurial unction, and of the method purſued; yet I am not clear in my opinion, whether the *ſaliva* of a mad cow, bitten
by a mad dog, would tranſmit the ſame vitiated *virus*, and poiſonous effects, to the perſons ſhe bit: for, poſſibly, the particles of the
mad dog's *ſaliva*, circulating in the blood of
the cow, might have the baneful effect of
producing fever, *delirium*, convulſions, *hydrophobia*, and death; and yet the aceſcent diſ-
poſition of the fluids in the cow might ſo alter
the nature of the particles of the dog's *ſaliva*
circulating in them, that the effect of the
cow's *ſaliva*, upon the perſons ſhe bit, was not
irritating to produce the bad ſymptoms. And
may not this be a material difference between
granivorous and *carnivorous* animals? Be that
as it may, I would not hazard my patients to
this conjecture, which repeated obſervation can
only determine.

With regard to Mrs. MEHEW, as ſhe had
no wound, nor ſcratch, of any kind, wherein
the *ſaliva* of the cow could be admitted; my
treatment of her was merely cautious, to prevent any ill effect from ſwallowing the leaſt
part of the cow's *ſaliva*; but chiefly to guard
againſt the approach of hyſteric and nervous
diſorders, which the ſurprize and apprehen-
ſion ſhe was thrown into might have produced.
With this view, I did not chuſe to have her
blooded

blooded with the others; but, after the vomit, and during the courfe of the medicines, I directed the ufe of *antihyfteric*, nervous, and cordial compofitions, to be taken with thofe particular ones recommended for the diftemper arifing from the bite of the mad dog: and I all along, and ever fince have, affured her, that I did not believe fhe was infected by the cow's *faliva*, nor would feel the leaft bad effect from it.

CASE VI.

The CASE *of* FRANCIS RAY, *blackfmith, of* Little Swaffham, *in the county of* Cambridge. *Communicated by* CHARLES ALLIX, Esq.

ON *Tuefday* the 19th of *November*, 1754, one RAY, a poor man, of *Little Swaffham*, applied to Mr. ALLIX, begging fome fea water for the ufe of his fon, 22 years of age; who, being at work with a blackfmith at *Cambridge*, was there bitten by a mad dog, three weeks before. The wound, between the fore finger and thumb, being only fkin deep, and not in the leaft painful, the young man gave no attention to it, till, at the new moon, on the 14th of *November*, his hand began to fwell, and be painful, and continued daily increafing till the 18th, when he went home to his father's.

Mr. AL-

Mr. ALLIX, not expecting any benefit from his sea water, which was grown stale, sent the young man two doses of Doctor JAMES's fever powders, with directions to take one as soon as the sea water had done working, and the other at night. Soon after, Mr. ALLIX, recollecting he had Doctor JAMES's pamphlet, which related, in a letter to professor BOERHAAVE, the effects of mercurials, in such cases; he set out, at two o'clock in the afternoon, for *Cambridge*, to have the medicines prepared.

In his way, Mr. ALLIX called on the young man, and looked at the wound, which was not open, but much inflamed, and round it a circular swelling. He complained of great pain in the wound, darting up the arm; had convulsive catches in his limbs, and his eyes looked very wild, and staring. He felt great anxiety in his sleep, and had been very feverish.

The sea water came partly off his stomach quite clear, the remainder purged him. Doctor JAMES's powder also vomited and purged him. It brought off a great deal of green stinking bile, after which the fever was much abated.

Between seven and eight in the evening, Mr. ALLIX called at *Little Swaffham*, on his return from *Cambridge*, when the swelling was increased, the inflammation more intense, extending itself quite up the wrist, and part

of

of his fore arm ; and complained that the pain, which grew more violent, now ſhot to his heart.

The part was immediately rubbed with half a dram of the mercurial ointment. The ſecond doſe of Doctor JAMES's powder having been juſt given, although forbidden by Mr. ALLIX ; he could not give the poor man the *turpeth mineral* bolus.

The fever powder having operated in a milder manner than the former doſe, the young man fell into a breathing ſweat, and quiet ſleep, which held him the whole night : next morning, *Wedneſday* the 20th *November*, Mr. ALLIX found the ſwelling greatly abated, and the man's looks more compoſed. He then took one of the following boluſſes :

℞ *Turpeth. mineral. gr.* xij. *pulv. contra-yerv. comp.* ʒj. *theriac. andromach. q. ſ. m. ſ. bol.* iij.

It worked him violently, upwards and down-wards : in the afternoon he took one of Doc-tor MEAD's powders (a dram and a half of the *pulvis antilyſſus*). The wound and hand were anointed, and directions were given to repeat the rubbing in of the ointment, morn-ing and evening.

Thurſday, 21ſt, the ſwelling, and inflamma-tion, were almoſt gone. A ſecond *turpeth* bo-lus was taken, which wrought very briſkly ;

and

and Doctor MEAD's powder was given in the afternoon.

Friday, the 22d, he complained, at times, of the pains returning, which alarmed him much. He took a *turpeth* bolus in the morning, and repeated the ointment both in the morning and evening, which he was directed to apply, as often as the pain and inflammation were inclined to return.

Saturday, 23d, the swelling and inflammation were not to be seen, his mouth began to be sore, and he spit much. Mr. ALLIX desired he would take another *turpeth* bolus that evening, and the two remaining doses of the *pulvis antilyssus* at proper intervals, lessening the quantity of the ointment to be rubbed in, by degrees. Mr. ALLIX, going out of the country for a few days, left orders with RAY's father, in case a salivation should come on, or the pain and inflammation return, to apply to Mr. JENNINGS, apothecary in *Cambridge*.

Wednesday, the 27th, Mr. ALLIX returned to *Swaffham*, and called on the poor man, whom he found free from complaints, only weakened by the regimen he had followed. In this gentleman's absence, the family had been alarmed at a trifling return of the pain and inflammation. Mr. JENNINGS had been sent for, and only ordered an electary with *valerian*, in addition to what was before directed.

The

The swelling and inflammation being now entirely gone, Mr. ALLIX desired the man to use the mercurial ointment very sparingly, and leave it off by degrees; and recommended, as soon as possible, the use of the cold bath. About the 10th of *December*, the young man, and his father, called upon Mr. ALLIX, to thank him for his charitable assistance, and to let him know that young RAY was quite well, and returning to work.

Mr. ALLIX farther observes, that, notwithstanding the visible effects of the mercurial ointment, in removing the pain and inflammation on the first application, and abating the violence of the symptoms, before even the first *turpeth* bolus was taken; they, more than once, seemed inclined to return, but were removed again by a fresh application of the ointment.

The diet was chicken, or other fresh white meat, and a glass or two of Madeira wine made into negus, to keep up his spirits.

REMARKS.

This Case affords evident proofs of the effects arising from the putrid *saliva* of a mad dog, in autumn; the progress is also plainly to be traced: and had not Mr. ALLIX's kind assistance been applied in the very critical moment, there is no doubt but the severest symp-

toms

toms had foon followed, and the patient had loft his life.

It is to be obferved, that the fea water, although ftale, diluted the green tenacious bile, and carried part of it downwards. Doctor JAMES's powders ferved as vomits, which cleared the ftomach from the vitiated putrid bile, and took off fo much of the irritation as to permit the *turpeth* bolus to be given without increafing the inflammation. But before the firft *turpeth* bolus was taken, the young man's fever and fwelling had abated; he had fallen into a breathing fweat, and flept quietly the whole night, after the firft mercurial unction on the *Tuefday* evening. On *Wednefday* morning the patient's looks were compofed, and then he took the firft *turpeth* bolus; and on *Thurfday* the fwelling and inflammation were almoft gone before the fecond *turpeth* bolus was taken. On *Saturday* the young man's mouth became fore, and he fpit much; notwithftanding which, Mr. ALLIX directed the third *turpeth* bolus to be given, and the remaining two dofes of the *pulvis antilyffus*; fo that the falivary and urinary difcharges were encouraged to the utmoft: but, for fear of increafing the falivation too much, the ointment was ordered to be then rubbed in fparingly.

In Mr. ALLIX's abfence, Mr. JENNINGS, the apothecary, only gave the patient an
electary

electary chiefly compofed of *valerian*, on account of his low and weak ftate after the fpit-
ting.—And on the 10th of *December*, that is,
at the end of three weeks, the young man
was perfectly cured.

If any farther proof be neceffary, of the
mercurial ointment having effected this cure;
Mr. ALLIX has added a very ftrong teftimony,
by faying, that the fymptoms were, more than
once, inclined to return, but were as often
removed by the application of the mercurial
ointment.

C A S E VII.

IN *March*, 1759, Mr. LEWIS ALSOP, a
butcher, aged about thirty years, of a ro-
buft make, but phlegmatic conftitution, had
the calf of his leg much tore by the bite of a
mad dog. He went down, immediately, to
Lynn in *Norfolk*, where he bathed in the fea.
His wound healed without difficulty. About
the end of *March*, 1760, having opened fhop
at *Witton*, in the county of *Huntingdon*, he
complained, to feveral of his cuftomers, that
the calf of his leg was very painful, particularly at the change and full of the moon, at
which time he always appeared much dejected.

Being confulted, I advifed him to rub all
over the calf of the leg, but more particularly over the wound, a dram of the *un-*

guentum

guentum cæruleum fortius, morning and evening, during a week, and every fourth day to
take a purge of *manna,* and of the *bitter purging falts.* This method having fucceeded, I
recommended the repetition of it three days
before every new and full moon, and as long
after, during three months, taking care to
purge, to prevent a falivation; which in-
junction he carefully followed, in the months
of *May, June,* and *July,* following. In *Oc-
tober* Mr. ALSOP came to me, ill of an intermitting fever, for which I directed a vomit,
and the *Peruvian* bark, whereby it was foon
cured.

In *December* 1760, he called upon me, to
thank me for all my care; and told me, he
had been free from pain, or any complaint in
his leg, fome months, and fo he continued to
his death, which, as I am informed by Mr.
HUNT, his apothecary, affiftant to SIR THO-
MAS MACKWORTH, was occafioned by a putrid fever, which he contracted from a neighbour, whom he vifited in his laft moments,
and of which fever he alfo died, on the fif-
teenth day, *March* 7, 1761.

REMARKS.

From the periodical returns of the pain in
the part which had been wounded, it appears,
that the bathing in the fea had not carried
off the *virus;* but that it remained in the
blood.

blood. The ceſſation of the pain, after the firſt mercurial unction, ſhews the power that *mercury* has of driving the vitiated *ſaliva* out by ſome of the emunctories: and had not Mr. ALSOP been perfectly cured from the effects of the bite he received from the mad dog, it is more than probable, that, in his laſt illneſs, the ſymptoms, ariſing from the bite, would have appeared.

Upon the ſtricteſt inquiry, I do not find, that he had either the dread of water, or of dogs, or any converſation tending to ex-preſs the remembrance of his former accident; but only the ſymptoms uſually attend-ing fevers of the kind which proved fatal to him.

CONCLUSION.

THE foregoing confiderations afford the pleafing hopes, that this difeafe, hitherto fo terrible, and aggravated by the apprehenfions which attend it, may now become, like others, more certainly cured; and therefore much lefs dreaded than heretofore.

But, before I proceed to lay down the directions to be followed, taken from the obfervations I have related, it may not be amifs to inquire, Whether the general alarm, fpread all over the cities of *London* and *Weftminfter*, and parts adjacent, in 1760, and alfo in feveral other parts of *England*, was occafioned by any real caufe, which infected dogs, and produced that madnefs? or whether it was merely a panic which had feized the inhabitants of thofe places?

The winter of the year 1759 had been very mild, and open; the fpring of 1760 very forward: fcarce any fnow, or froft, had appeared in thofe feafons; and, during the whole fummer, myriads of infects were feen in every leaf, upon the trees; and the fprings, remarkably low, were full of them; more particularly the ditches, and pools of ftagnating waters, of which the cattle were frequently obliged to drink, through the fcarcity of water:

and

and even the inhabitants of feveral villages had no other fupply. Hence arofe, in the autumn, efpecially among the poorer fort of people, putrid fevers, of fuch a malignant nature, as to be little inferior to peftilential diftempers. Perfons, in all appearance, in ftrength, and vigor of health, were carried off, in three, five, feven, or nine days, with the moft violent marks of malignity and putrefaction. All had *petechiæ*; and none efcaped without critical abfceffes of the *axillary*, *inguinal*, and fometimes of the *parotid* glands.

No wonder, then, that the brute creation were alfo liable to fuch illnefs as corrupted waters could bring on; and efpecially if their food was equally corrupt, which dogs are known to feed upon of choice. The offals, ufually caft about the fhambles in every great town; the ftinking waters contained in fome marfhy grounds; and, perhaps, even the want of water, in many places, might caufe this madnefs among the dogs.

It firft appeared in the borough of *Southwark*; and the confternation diffufed itfelf all over the cities of *London* and *Weftminfter*. The magiftrates immediately iffued out a very prudent and judicious order, for every perfon, who kept dogs, to confine them, during a month, within doors; and ordered their beadles, and other officers, to deftroy all dogs found at large; with a reward of two fhillings for each dog which fhould be killed.

But

But as the wifeft and moft judicious intentions are frequently perverted, and the moft
beneficial regulations prove oppreffive, through
an abufe of power; fo this reward prompted
a licentious rabble to kill every dog they could
meet, within their reach, with all the barba-
rity poffible: and too, often the number of
real mad dogs was increafed, by the violent
purfuits and attacks of the giddy and unthink-
ing populace. Therefore it muft appear very
plain, that, as there was fufficient caufe, in
that hot feafon, to produce the putrid fever,
and madnefs, among dogs; fo their number
was multiplied, by the barbarous ufage they
met with; and even all thefe added, fell far
fhort, in number, to thofe who were killed
through wantonnefs, and without reafon.

The fatal perfuafion, that there was no cure
for the difeafe incident to mankind from the
bite of a mad dog, may have juftified the
confternation which was fo general in the metropolis: but now, that, in many parts of the
world, fuccefsful cures have fhewn this malady not to be incurable, there can be no longer
any plea for that extreme anxiety and fear.

There is but one general rule to be obferved
in the treatment of this diforder, that is, the
application of the *mercurial ointment*, which
can never be fafely difpenfed with: all other
rules, of evacuations, external applications,
or internal medicines, muft be varied, according to the ftage of the difeafe, the age, and
con-

conftitution, of the patient. However, for the direction of fuch who may not be at hand to have affiftance, the following particulars are mentioned.

The part bitten fhould immediately be cleaned from the *faliva* of the mad dog, and the wounds encouraged to bleed, carefully clearing the blood away; then half a dram of the *mercurial ointment*, known by the name of *unguentum cæruleum fortius*, or the *ftronger blue ointment*, fhould be rubbed in, and repeated night and morning, increafing or leffening the quantity, as it may prove neceffary. Sanguine conftitutions will require bleeding; leucophlegmatic, relaxed, and bilious ones, fhould be vomited, either with *ipecacuanha* wine, with or without *oxymel of fquills*, which will cleanfe the ftomach and bowels from the putrid bile, and acrid *faliva*, that has been difcharged into them; and in the advanced ftage, when liquids begin to pafs with difficulty, if it be requifite to empty the ftomach and bowels, after plentiful bleedings, fome grains of *ipecacuanha* and *white hellebore* root may be given in a bolus, made up with the *oxymel of fquills*. Thefe vomits will be lefs apt to irritate the *primæ viæ*, than either *turpeth mineral*, or any *antimonial* preparation.

Doctor MEAD's *pulvis antilyffus* may then be taken every morning, in warm milk, to procure the urinary difcharges, while the *mercurial* frictions are continued; and if thefe are
inclined

inclined to falivate, an emollient clyfter; or a purge, with *manna, cooling falts,* and *rhubarb,* may be given. *Rhubarb,* either in powder, or the fyrup, will be beft adapted to children. Clyfters are recommended, in all ftages, by Doctor DESAULT, profeffor BOERHAAVE, and Doctor MEAD; and are to be compofed of fuch ingredients as the cafe may require, whether emollient, or coolers. After the mercurial ointment has been ufed four or five days, and the patient purged with fome of the abovementioned medicines, or, if neceffary, with *crude mercury,* divided with *turpentine,* and mixed with *rhubarb,* or by *mercurius dulcis,* well fublimed, and mixed with *rhubarb;* then it may be proper, in fome cafes, efpecially where the fpafms are frequent, to give the *cinnabars,* either with or without *muſk,* as perfumes agree or difagree with the patient: indeed there are inftances wherein *muſk* has not been difagreeable to the ftomach, although the perfon could not ufually bear the fmell of it. The *cinnabar* powders are to be taken every fix or eight hours, with a julep of *rue water, pennyroyal water, tincture of caftor,* and fome common fyrup, or in a glafs of *arrack* alone, or with water.

In tender conftitutions, antifpafmodic and antihyfteric medicines may be ufed, towards the end of the cure; but nature, in this difeafe, no more than in any acute diforder, is not to be overcharged with medicines: for,

as

as Doctor M O R T O N obferves *, " an officious
" overloading feldom goes off unpunifhed."
And care muft be taken, left, inftead of
ftrengthening the nerves, they fuffer not by
too much irritation.

Such patients as can, without fear, be prevailed upon to go into the cold bath, willingly
and of themfelves, may complete their cure
by that immerfion; but force, or too earneft
perfuafion, are cautioufly to be avoided.

The diet to be kept, during the mercurial
frictions, which, as hath been faid, are to be
repeated according to the cafe, and intirely depended upon, is to be light and nourifhing,
neither high feafoned, nor acrid : in the worft
ftages, a moderate quantity of wine may increafe the inflammation; whereas wine may
be of ufe in the beginning, and in a dejected
ftate. White meats will fuit the ftomach
beft; and milk pottage, water gruel, *polenta*,
that is, a decoction of *oatbread* toafted, and
toaft and water, may be drank : as likewife an
infufion of *black currants* ftalks and leaves, or
baum tea fweetned with *black currant* jelly :
thefe two laft will better fuit in the inflamma-
tory ftage.

So far from confining the patients to their
room, or houfe; exercife, company, and di-
verfions, are to be encouraged : for the mind

* Natura non debet laceffi medicamentis. Quod fit
officiofe raro impune patratur. RICHARDI MORTON
Exercitationes.

being

being as much affected as the body, the cure will be much forwarded by a proper application to the paffions, avoiding all converfation relating to madnefs, or mad dogs. Doctor Desault relates * the fuccefs which attended thefe directions which he gave to a lady of *Bourdeaux*, who, under the courfe of mercurial frictions, conftantly vifited her friends, went to concerts, and other public places.

Thus far the cure is only preventive of the *hydrophobia*, and defigned for the milder progrefs of the difeafe, and alfo when it is complicated with *hypochondriac* or *hyfterical* fymptoms; but in the confirmed ftate, when the *hydrophobia* appears, the actual cure is to be performed by copious and repeated bleedings, cooling clyfters, often adminiftred, of *barley water, nitre, honey, and vinegar;* and, after thefe evacuations, it may be allowable, in cafe of a confiderable flow of the *faliva*, to apply a blifter round the neck, to take off part of the difcharge, as fucceeded in Doctor Hele's remarkable obfervation: this is the only time wherein blifters can be fafely applied.—But the medicine chiefly to be depended upon is the *mercurial ointment*, which is to be rubbed in three times a day, and continued till the fymptoms decreafe, and the difcharge from the glands of the mouth

---

* Desault Differtation fur la rage, p. 311.

fhew

ſhew it is proper to leſſen the quantity of the ointment.

When the throat and ſtomach will admit of liquids, the ſame method, above mentioned, may be purſued, towards compleating the cure.

F I N I S.

Publiſhed by the ſame AUTHOR.

I. An ESSAY on the Contagious Diſtemper among the Horned Cattle.

II. A DISCOURSE on the Uſefulneſs of Inoculating the Horned Cattle. Read before the *Royal Society.*